A Woman's Guide
to Living with HIV Infection

A Johns Hopkins Press Health Book

A Woman's Guide to Living with HIV Infection

Rebecca A. Clark, M.D., Ph.D.

Robert T. Maupin, Jr., M.D., FACOG

Jill Hayes Hammer, Ph.D.

THE JOHNS HOPKINS UNIVERSITY PRESS
Baltimore & London

Note to the reader: *This book is not meant to substitute for medical care. Treatment plans for people with HIV infection must be developed in a dialogue between an individual and her primary care provider. Our book is intended to help with that dialogue.*

Drug dosage: *The author and publisher have made reasonable efforts to determine that the selection and dosage of drugs discussed in this text conform to the actual practices of the general medical community. However, the medications described do not necessarily have specific approval by the U.S. Food and Drug Administration for use in the diseases and dosages for which they are recommended here. In view of ongoing research, changes in governmental regulations, and the constant flow of information relating to drug therapy and drug reactions, the reader is urged to check the package insert of each drug for any change in indications and dosage and for warnings and precautions. This is particularly important when the recommended agent is a new and/or infrequently used drug.*

The authors acknowledge and appreciate thoughtful reviews of selected chapters by Mary Murphy, M.D. (chapter 5), Marsha J. Bennett, D.N.S., A.P.R.N., A.C.R.N. (chapter 19), Harlee Kutzen, M.N., A.C.R.N. (chapter 17), and Jan Vick, L.C.S.W. (chapter 18).

© 2004 The Johns Hopkins University Press

The Johns Hopkins University Press
2715 North Charles Street
Baltimore, Maryland 21218-4363
www.press.jhu.edu

Library of Congress Cataloging-in-Publication Data

Clark, Rebecca A., 1958–
   A woman's guide to living with HIV infection / Rebecca A. Clark,
Robert T. Maupin Jr., Jill Hayes Hammer.
      p.   cm. — (A Johns Hopkins Press health book)
Includes bibliographical references and index.
   ISBN 0-8018-7913-2 (hardcover : alk. paper)—ISBN 0-8018-7914-0
(pbk. : alk. paper)
   1. HIV-positive women—Medical care.   2. AIDS (Disease) in women.
3. HIV infections.   4. Women—Health and hygiene.   I. Maupin,
Robert T., 1963–   II. Hammer, Jill Hayes, 1968–   III. Title.   IV. Series.
   RC607.A26C5685 2004
   362.196′9792′0082—dc22   2003017427

A catalog record for this book is available from the British Library.

This book is dedicated to women living with HIV,
in recognition of their courage and the challenges many of them overcome
to obtain care for themselves and their children.

Contents

A Woman's Guide
to Living with HIV Infection

Introduction:
Women and the HIV/AIDS Epidemic

What is the Human Immunodeficiency Virus?

What is the history of the HIV/AIDS epidemic?

What is the best way to read this book?

First, some comforting facts:

- *You are not alone.* Every year, thousands of women in the United States are diagnosed with HIV.
- HIV infections have been reported in every area in the United States, even in very small towns in the countryside.
- Anyone who has ever had sex could have become infected with HIV. This includes the vast majority of adults. You need not feel embarrassed that you are infected.
- Current HIV treatments are extremely powerful. If you have not been sick from your HIV infection, there is a good chance that you may never get sick. If you are sick, it is likely that you can get better, particularly if you are starting HIV treatments for the first time.

We have written this guide to help you understand HIV and to help you find support and treatment for yourself or for the woman with HIV in your life. HIV stands for "human immunodeficiency virus." It differs from other viruses like cold viruses because, unlike most other viral infections, HIV damages people's immune systems—the complex defense network that our bodies rely on to protect us from infections of all kinds. People infected with HIV who do not receive treatment eventually lose their natural ability to defend themselves from infections. AIDS (which stands for "Acquired Immune Deficiency Syndrome") means that the immune system of someone who is infected with HIV has lost the ability to prevent medical conditions that other people rarely experience. Today, thanks to new medications that hold HIV in check, AIDS is an avoidable and treatable condition. One of the goals of this book is to explain the power of these highly effective medications.

The HIV/AIDS epidemic currently affects hundreds of thousands of women in the United States and around the world. Approximately 50 percent of adults living with HIV or AIDS worldwide are women. At the beginning of the epidemic, men were thought to be at higher risk than women for developing AIDS, but AIDS is now recognized as a growing problem among women. The Centers for Disease Control and Prevention (CDC), an agency in the U.S. Department of Health and Human Services, has monitored the number of cases of AIDS in the United States since 1986 when the epidemic first appeared among gay men. Soon after, people who used injectable street drugs or who received blood products were also found to be at risk for HIV infection.

Initially, less than 5 percent of the AIDS cases recorded by the CDC were women. This low number suggests either that HIV infection was uncommon among women at the beginning or that health care providers were simply not recognizing AIDS in women with symptoms. Since the mid-1980s, however, more and more women have developed unmistakable AIDS. In the year 2001, 26 percent of the recorded new AIDS cases were in women, and the CDC estimates that 30 percent of the approximately 40,000 new HIV infections that occur each year in the United States are in women. Since 1996, an average of 10,500 cases of AIDS have been diagnosed in American women each year, and an estimated 25 percent of the 850,000 to 950,000 of those living with HIV/AIDS in the United States are women.

HIV has disproportionately affected women of color. In the United States 64 percent of the female cases in 2001 were among African-American women (nearly twenty-three times higher than the rate among Caucasian women), and 17 percent of the female cases in 2001 were among Hispanic women (more than five times higher than the rate among Caucasian women).

Most women with HIV were infected by having sex with men. Although approximately 2 percent of the women diagnosed with AIDS have identified themselves as having sex with women, nearly all of them had other risk factors for HIV, so it is likely that they acquired HIV, not by having sex with other women, but by some other means. Clearly, for women, sex with men—heterosexual sex—is the number-one risk factor for acquiring HIV. The second major risk factor is using injectable street drugs.

We wrote this book for women personally affected by HIV/AIDS as well as for their families and friends. Other books that provide medical information about HIV do not comprehensively cover topics of special interest to women, and most books on women's health do not discuss women with HIV. Yet women with HIV have unique concerns regarding gynecologic disorders, reproductive choices, contraception, and pregnancy. We believe this book will help many women to lead better informed and, we hope, healthier lives.

How to Read This Book

You can read this book all at once, or you can read the parts that are of special concern to you right now. Some women diagnosed with HIV immediately want to get as much information about the infection as they can. Others prefer to learn more gradually over time. Our goal is to help you stay as healthy as you can, so whichever way you choose to approach the information, we have included what you need to know to work with your health care providers at a comfortable pace. Table I.1 outlines the major topics covered in this guide.

Table I.1

Topics Covered in *A Woman's Guide to Living with HIV Infection*

HIV-Related Health Issues
  Description of how HIV affects women's bodies
  HIV-related medical conditions among women
  Treatments for HIV and its related conditions
  Preventing HIV-related complications

General Health Issues
  Gynecologic topics
  Health maintenance
  Mental health

Reproduction and Contraception
  Reproductive choices
  Birth control options
  Pregnancy

How to Make the Health Care System Work for You
  Finding a testing site
  Finding a primary care provider
  Various resources
  Assistance programs

Miscellaneous
  Clinical trial and study participation
  Chronic pain
  Substance use
  Abusive relationships

This book provides information on the medical, emotional, and social issues facing women with HIV infection. It also explores women's general health issues, answering the kinds of questions that many of our patients ask us. Each chapter begins with key questions and ends with key points.

When discussing drugs, we use two names: the brand name (also known as the trade name), and the scientific name (also known as the generic name) of the drug. For example, Retrovir is the brand name for the generic drug called zidovudine. They are exactly the same medicine. Some chapters include a list of useful resources, including Web sites. There are two appendixes. The first is a "medication, test, and vaccine tracking sheet" for use by patients, and the second is a list of helpful Web sites and phone resources. A glossary at the end of the book provides brief definitions of medical terms. Finally, a list of selected scientific references is also available at the end of the book.

We urge women with HIV/AIDS to become as informed as possible and to seek medical care and treatment. Our purpose is to help women avoid HIV-related complications like sickness, sadness, isolation, and confusion. Reading this medical guide can prepare you for clinic visits and can help make these visits more productive for both you and your health care provider. Sometimes it is hard to remember everything you have heard in a clinic visit; this book will help you remember and understand information you may not have fully processed the first time around.

If you have HIV, you need to know that you have a chronic yet treatable condition that can often be controlled. By reading this book, you are taking a positive step toward improving your health. Here you will learn what is happening to your body. You will learn how to prevent HIV-related complications, and you will learn about treatment.

KEY POINTS

1. Approximately one-fourth of the 850,000 to 950,000 Americans living with HIV or AIDS are women.

2. Women make up an increasing proportion of the AIDS cases reported to the Centers for Disease Control.

3. The rates of HIV infection are higher among African-American and Hispanic women than among white women.

4. *In most cases, women acquire HIV infection by having sex with HIV-infected men.*

5. *In this book, we explain what HIV does to women's bodies; we describe HIV-related medical conditions in women; we explore issues related to reproduction and contraception for women with HIV; and we describe the treatment available to women with HIV.*

PART ONE

Adjusting to Life with HIV Infection

Millions of people today are living with HIV. What was once a very mysterious disease has become a familiar diagnosis in America and around the world. In the past twenty-five years, researchers have made fantastic gains in understanding and treating HIV. New medications are now turning this once-deadly disease into a chronic and manageable one. But HIV is not a diagnosis anyone takes lightly. Adjusting to life with HIV requires effort and patience. It will most likely affect how you feel, how you manage your health, and how you choose to live. HIV is a disease that requires lifelong monitoring, but it is no longer a disease of utter mystery and terror.

1

Testing for HIV

What tests are used to diagnose HIV infection?

How soon do these tests turn positive after a person has been infected with HIV?

Where should a person go for testing?

How will you feel if you receive a positive test result?

Who should you tell about your test results?

ELISA and Western Blot Testing

The most common test for the human immunodeficiency virus (or "HIV test") is a blood test that looks for antibodies to HIV. An antibody is a protein that the body makes to fight infection. The HIV test does not look for actual HIV in the blood. Instead, it looks for the antibodies to HIV. It recognizes your body's reaction to the virus.

Antibodies cannot be detected the instant a person is infected because it takes two to eight weeks from the time the virus first infects a person's blood for the body to mount a full antibody response. *Infected blood tested for antibodies during the first weeks after exposure to HIV will return a negative result: the test will look negative for antibodies even though the blood is infected with HIV.* This means that if your test results are negative one month after an exposure, you may actually have HIV, but your body has not yet made detectable antibodies. To ensure accuracy of the test result, a second HIV test is recommended for three months after exposure and, depending on the type of exposure, a third test may be advised for six months after exposure. Over 95 percent of people with HIV have a positive HIV test by three months after they are infected, and over 99 percent have a positive test by six months.

There are two standard antibody tests: the ELISA and the Western blot. The ELISA test is done first. If the ELISA is positive, then the Western blot test is performed (using the same blood sample) to confirm the result of the ELISA. These tests may yield different results. The ELISA test will either be positive or negative, but the Western blot test can be positive, negative, or indeterminate (which means the test results are inconclusive). If you have a positive ELISA and negative Western blot test, you are assumed to be HIV-negative. If your ELISA and Western blot tests are both positive, you are assumed to have HIV. But if your ELISA is positive and your Western blot is indeterminate, your HIV infection status is still unclear. You may be negative, or you may be in the process of making detectable antibodies (a process called "seroconverting"). Generally repeat testing after three months is recommended to clarify the answer. If you are consistently indeterminate on your Western blot and you have no clear risk factors for becoming infected with HIV, you are probably negative. Sometimes viral load testing (as described in chapter 4) or polymerase chain reaction testing (see below) will help define your status if you repeatedly

Table 1.1
How to Interpret HIV Test Results

ELISA	Western blot	True HIV status
positive	positive	positive
positive	negative	negative
positive	indeterminate	unclear*
negative	not done	negative

* Repeat testing is necessary. See text for explanation.

receive an indeterminate Western blot result. Table 1.1 summarizes these different test result combinations.

Other HIV Screening Tests

Some testing centers are now using a saliva test called Orasure, which does not require an injection. If the Orasure test is positive, you should have a confirmatory test with the ELISA (and if the ELISA is positive, you should have a Western blot test).

There are also rapid tests generally used in hospital settings that give results within 30 minutes. Again, positive results need to be confirmed with additional testing.

How Accurate Are the Tests?

The Orasure test is more than 99 percent accurate. The chance that the ELISA and Western blot test are both wrong is extremely small—less than 1 in 100,000. However, it is possible (although very unlikely) that your first screening could be wrong. If you have any doubts about the result, you should have the test repeated. For example, if you know you were exposed to HIV infection and yet you received negative results, or if, on the other hand, you do not think you have any risk factors for HIV infection and yet you received a positive result—then you should have another HIV test.

Screening Test in Infants

Tests used for infants are different from those used for adults. A polymerase chain reaction (PCR) test, which detects the genetic material of HIV, is not routinely used to screen adults but it is often used to check whether newborn infants have HIV.

The antibody tests (the ELISA and Western blot) are not the best tests to use for screening infants because a mother's antibodies pass through the placenta to the baby and stay in the baby's blood for up to 15 months. This means that if the mother is HIV-infected, then her baby's antibody test may be positive from birth until the child is 15 months old even if the baby does not have HIV. For this reason, infants' blood should be tested for the actual presence of HIV, not for presence of the antibody.

If a baby's PCR test is positive, it is likely that the baby is truly infected. Unfortunately, a negative PCR result is not 100 percent reliable. An HIV culture is sometimes done to help determine whether an infant is infected (HIV can be cultured in special laboratories). Yet it is possible for an HIV-infected infant to have both a negative PCR and a negative culture. If these tests are negative, they should be repeated. If the tests remain negative for up to three months, the infant probably is HIV-negative but should still have additional follow-up testing. The usual schedule of testing involves four PCR tests: the first at birth, the second at three to six weeks, the third at six to twelve weeks, and the fourth at twelve to twenty-four months. An ELISA test is done between 15 and 18 months of age.

Procedures for HIV Testing and Reporting

Every testing center should offer pre-test and post-test counseling to explain what the tests mean. If you are looking for a test center, ask whether they offer pre-test and post-test counseling, and try to choose a center that does. The counselors will explain how to decrease the risk of becoming infected with HIV if you are found to be HIV-negative and how to decrease the risk of transmitting the virus if you are found to have HIV. If you have HIV, counselors will let you know how you can receive medical treatment if needed. They will also answer your questions. Almost everyone has questions, and it is very important for you to get the expert answers you need. This means having focused and confidential time to talk to counselors. The points covered in pre-test and post-test counseling are listed in table 1.2.

There are two ways to have an HIV test done: anonymous testing and confidential testing. *Anonymous testing* means there is no possibility of connecting the person who was tested with the result of the test through any identifier such as name, Social Security number, or hospi-

Table 1.2

Points Covered in Pre-test and Post-test Counseling

Pre-test Counseling

- General information about HIV, including how HIV is transmitted and what happens to your body with HIV infection
- What positive, negative, and indeterminate HIV test results mean
- What a confidential or anonymous HIV test means
- Importance of coming back for the results and what type of follow-up can be expected if the test is positive or indeterminate
- How to decrease the risk of acquiring HIV
- Referrals to other services if needed
- A consent to do the test

Post-test Counseling

The discussion of test results will depend on your status:

- Negative: Discuss again how HIV is transmitted and how you can decrease the risk; discuss whether and when to get a repeat test
- Indeterminate: Discuss what the test means and the need for repeat testing
- Positive: Discuss the difference between having HIV and having AIDS; referral to the appropriate clinics and services; discuss how to decrease the risk of transmitting the infection to others

Source: Adapted from J. Anderson, ed., *A Guide to the Clinical Care of Women with HIV.* U.S. Department of Health and Human Services, Health Resources Services Administration at http://www.hrsa.gov/hab, table 3.2.

tal number. With anonymous testing, the tested person is usually given a number, and the results are linked to that number. You are asked to read and sign a consent form for the HIV test, but "signing" in this case means writing in the number you have been assigned or signing an "X"; it does not mean writing your actual name. When the results are available, you give your number to get your results. If you choose to receive anonymous testing, your test result will not appear in your medical records.

Another way to have an HIV test done is through *confidential testing.* Confidential HIV testing does use an identifier to link the results to the person tested. This means that the test results will be placed in your medical record. The results should only be available to the medical staff taking care of you and to the medical insurance company covering your medical care. Nonmedical persons would have to get a court order to see your medical chart. With confidential testing, you will be asked to read and sign a consent form to have the HIV test.

Public health offices need to keep careful and accurate records regarding epidemic diseases like HIV and AIDS. State health departments require the reporting of every case of AIDS, and some also require reporting of HIV. This information is gathered to help direct resources most effectively to people in need. Many people are concerned about the privacy of their medical records. Offices of public health take confidentiality very seriously; there are multiple safeguards in place to prevent wrongful access to personal information.

Most cities offer free HIV testing at various locations. You can also get the confidential test through a doctor's office, but not the anonymous test. Before you select a testing location, think about whether you want an anonymous or a confidential test, find out whether pre-test and post-test counseling is available, and find out if there is a charge for the test (and, if so, what the charge will be).

Feelings about a Positive Test

Different people react in different ways when they learn they have been infected with HIV. Disbelief is a very common reaction, especially for people who thought they were not at risk for HIV. Some HIV-positive women continue for a very long time to deny that they could have HIV. The reality of the epidemic is that most women acquire their HIV infection through sex, yet many women with HIV have *not* had many sexual partners. After disbelief, a subsequent emotion is anger. You may be angry at the unfairness of the situation, and you may also be angry with the person you think infected you.

Many people also feel depression or despair or panic. You may be concerned about whether you already have AIDS and whether your life will be shortened. These are common first reactions; learning more about this disease and its excellent prospects for treatment often helps

Table 1.3
Strategies for Coping with a New HIV Diagnosis

1. Educate yourself and learn about your condition. You may be reassured.
2. Share information about your condition with family and friends you feel comfortable with. Do not isolate yourself.
3. Other sources of support may include your church or other community organizations. Many community organizations that help people with HIV have support groups that meet regularly to allow people to share experiences, joys, and frustrations.
4. If you feel very depressed or anxious, consider talking with a mental health provider such as a psychologist, psychiatrist, or social worker. Seeking help for your feelings makes sense and does not mean you are "crazy." Many people have emotional difficulty after learning they have a chronic disease.
5. Take good care of yourself by following the guidelines described on page 36.
6. Keep busy. If you are not employed outside the home and you don't work at home taking care of children, consider volunteer opportunities. Activity is important.
7. Take time to do things you enjoy.

to ease these feelings. Depression is described in chapter 16. You may fear the unknown and feel poorly informed about your own medical condition and about possible HIV treatments—this is true for many people. If you are pregnant, you may fear for the health of your unborn baby. Sometimes what people feel is not fear but anxiety. Anxiety is also discussed in chapter 16. Other typical responses include fear of separation from your partner and concern about what will happen to people who depend on you, should you become sick. Strategies for coping with these feelings are listed in table 1.3.

Who Should You Tell?

Keeping HIV a secret can be a tremendous burden, particularly if you are taking HIV treatments and feel the need to hide your medications. Still, some women are reluctant to disclose their HIV status because they are afraid the information will drive their friends and family away or make them worry. But friends and family can be very supportive— often surprisingly so. Many women report that their families responded with much more strength and encouragement than they had expected.

It is very important to let your sexual partner or partners know your test results. If you are uncomfortable explaining by yourself, ask a friend or family member to be there to support you. If you are afraid of how your partner may react, you may want to deliver the news indirectly. One option is to have your primary care provider contact your partner to discuss the results. Many public health sexually transmitted disease clinics will send a letter to a partner without giving specific information that would provide a clue about who was tested. For example, the letter can tell a partner that he or she was exposed to a sexually transmitted disease within the last ten years. Fear of telling a partner in person may be well justified, because women sometimes face a real risk of abuse from a partner after disclosure. Abuse can be physical, emotional, or verbal (dealing with abuse is discussed in chapter 15).

The decision whether or not to tell your children—and how much to tell—will depend on their ages. Table 1.4 summarizes the level of understanding to expect from children at different developmental stages. If you are sick and have frequent clinic visits or if you are admitted to the hospital, it is probably better to share as much as you comfortably can. Children have powerful imaginations, and very often their fears are much worse than the situation warrants. Some of their main fears are going to be about who will take care of them if you are sick and what will happen to them. They may be reassured if you talk things over with them.

Whoever you share your diagnosis with will probably want more information. If you are comfortable bringing family members with you to your clinic visits, your health care provider will probably welcome the opportunity to discuss any questions they may have, as long as you approve. If you would rather not involve other people during your appointments, you can refer friends and family to one of the many

Table 1.4
How Much Can a Child Understand Illness at Different Ages?

Developmental stage	
Infants and toddlers (0–2)	• Infants and toddlers will have little or no understanding of what is going on, but they are uniquely in tune with you. They experience your emotions as if they were their own. If you are upset, they are upset. • Also, children may become anxious and fearful if the parent becomes withdrawn or is unresponsive to their needs.
Pre-school (2–6)	• Children at this age will not understand the concept of disease, but they will understand what it means to be "sick." Their biggest concern will likely be how your sickness will affect them. • If you decide to disclose your illness to your child, it would be comforting to focus on the fact that while you are sick, you will try your best to make sure that your child's life will remain as normal as possible. Disruptions in daily routines and changes in caregivers can shake a child's sense of trust. • Even though they can talk, most children up to about four years of age communicate a great deal through their play. For example, if a child is upset, she may act it out through her play. It is helpful to watch your child's play for clues about her feelings.
School-age (6–10)	• Children at this age level develop both independence and cognitive skills fairly quickly. They likely understand concepts like death and disease, though they may have some misconceptions about these issues. Friends or television may be the source of incorrect information.

(continued)

Table 1.4 (*continued*)

Developmental stage	
	For example, the child may think that if you have HIV, you are going to die.
	• For this reason, children at this age benefit from accurate information, but they can also be overwhelmed by too much information. Be brief. Give the child some information, and then let her ask questions. Take her lead in deciding how much information to give, and be patient. Questions may come right away, or they may come after the child has had time to process the information.
	• It may be a good idea to distract the child with fun activities because at this age it still may be difficult for a child to handle too much too quickly.
	• Children at this age often can put themselves in your shoes and may feel bad for you. At the same time, they may also be angry with you. They may blame you for getting HIV. Young children tend to see things as black and white.
Early adolescence (girls 10–13; boys 12–15)	• Children understand death and disease at this age. They will likely know something is going on even if you decide not to tell them your diagnosis. If you decide to share information about your situation with your pre-adolescent child, an accurate portrayal of what is going on with you is necessary. Still, don't give them too much nonessential detail. Honestly answer their questions.
	• Be aware of what is going on with your child as well. Early adolescence is a time of rapid physical change and mood swings.
	• If a young adolescent is upset or anxious, he may show how upset he is through aggression,

Table 1.4 (*continued*)

Developmental stage	
	sleep problems, crying spells, or physical symptoms like headaches and upset stomach.
Adolescence (13–18)	• Adolescents understand death and disease. Disclosure to them must be accurate but not too full of details unless the adolescent asks questions.
	• Adolescents also are on an emotional and hormonal roller coaster. They may act out their emotions through aggression, experimentation with drugs and sex, or poor school performance, and they may become more defiant.
	• A contradiction in behavior is also normal at this age: the teen may love and hate the same person at the same time, for example; and while she craves independence, she also wants dependable structure in her life. Security is important to adolescents; having a parent with a disease can threaten this security.

HIV/AIDS organizations that offer support groups. Some organizations have groups specifically for women. In a support group, you may find comfort in learning how other women told their families and how their families reacted. Responses vary. Negative reactions are often due to misinformation and lack of information.

KEY POINTS

1. The two tests that are usually used to screen for HIV are the ELISA and the Western blot. These tests screen for HIV antibodies.

2. Generally the antibody screening tests will be positive by three months after a person is infected.

3. *There is a saliva test (Orasure) that can screen for HIV; a positive test should be confirmed by the blood antibody tests.*

4. *A test that checks for genetic material of the HIV is called a polymerase chain reaction (PCR) test. It is usually used to test infants born to HIV-infected mothers.*

5. *Every center that does HIV testing should offer pre- and post-test counseling.*

6. *The results of any HIV test should always be confidential; some centers offer anonymous testing.*

7. *When people first learn they have HIV, common reactions include disbelief, denial, anger, depression, and anxiety.*

2

Finding a Primary Care Provider and Preparing for Your Visit

What should you look for when you choose a primary care provider?

What should you expect at the first office visit or clinic visit?

What should you expect at follow-up office visits or clinic visits?

Finding a Primary Care Provider

One of the most important services an HIV testing center can provide is referral to a good primary care provider who has a great deal of experience taking care of people infected with HIV. Generally, a counselor at the testing site will give you the name, phone number, and address of an internist or infectious disease specialist who works in connection with a multiservice HIV clinic. Other physicians such as obstetrician/gynecologists and family practitioners also frequently care for people with HIV. Nurse practitioners and physician assistants may be excellent primary care providers as well.

Research has shown that you will have a better chance of staying

Table 2.1
How to Choose a Primary Care Provider or Clinic

Look for the following services:

Social work and case management services: Social workers and case managers can assist with transportation, housing, benefits, and disability issues. Your clinic provider should have links to these resources or be able to refer you to them.

Nutritional services: Nutritional complications can be associated with HIV. A clinic-associated nutritionist can assist with counseling or obtaining nutritional supplements if needed.

Mental health care: Your HIV primary care provider should have links to mental health services.

Gynecological care: If your Pap smears can be done by your primary care provider, you will not need to make a separate clinic appointment to have this test done.

Obstetrical care: There should be established coordination between HIV primary care and obstetrical services.

Pediatric care: If a clinic offers joint appointments for you and your child, you will not need to make two visits.

Eye care: If your HIV disease is advanced, you will need regular eye exams. There should be established coordination between HIV primary care and eye services.

Dental care: Dental problems are very common and can lead to complications such as weight loss. If dental care is not provided on site, there should be established coordination between HIV primary care and dental services.

Subspecialty services: Subspecialties such as neurology, infectious diseases, hematology/oncology, endocrinology, and pulmonary are often needed. There should be established coordination between these services and HIV primary care.

Medication availability: Medications may be available in some clinics through samples from drug companies, patient assistance programs, and grants for uninsured patients.

Table 2.1 *(continued)*

Research opportunities: If studies of HIV treatments are done in the clinic, you can avoid visiting two different locations.

Clinic availability after routine hours: If the clinic offers evenings or weekend appointments, you may not need to miss work or school.

Accommodation for urgent appointments: If a clinic leaves time available each day for urgent appointments, you may avoid emergency room visits.

Availability of assistance after hours: If there is assistance after hours by phone, you may avoid emergency room visits.

healthy if you receive care from an experienced provider who has taken care of other people with HIV or AIDS. However, if you have a good relationship with a primary care provider who lacks experience managing HIV, you may still want to continue seeing that person. Together, you and your primary care provider can find an HIV specialist who will act as a consultant for your HIV treatment.

If more than one clinic or provider is available to you, there are several questions to consider when making your choice. These are listed in table 2.1. Recognizing how burdensome it is for patients to travel to different locations for appointments, some clinics provide "one-stop shopping" by gathering several needed specialties together at the same site. You may need to decide if you want to travel a longer distance to visit a clinic with more services, or whether you prefer a closer, though more limited clinic.

What to Expect at the First Visit

You may feel nervous when scheduling your first clinic visit. After all, you are setting out on an unfamiliar path. It may be helpful to remember that the health care team waiting to meet you at the clinic is devoted to your health and well-being. A number of different people will want to meet with you, so the first visit will take some time. You will also have a number of tests, and this too can take time. When you call to schedule your first clinic appointment, you may want to ask how long it will take. The person scheduling the appointment should also tell you what information you need to bring with you, such as personal identification and information regarding your health insurance, if you have it, and your financial status (for example, a pay stub or a statement from the unemployment office).

Try to get to bed early the night before your first appointment. In the morning, eat a healthy breakfast with plenty of fluids. The first appointment can be tiring, but it can also give you strength by introducing you to the team of dedicated experts who will follow your health closely and who will be available to help you whenever you have questions or concerns.

At the first visit, you should expect to have several tubes of blood drawn for various tests. These tests include "routine" laboratory tests (called "labs") that check your blood count, blood sugar, kidney function, and liver function as well as special labs that check your HIV infection. (Chapter 4 explains the nature of HIV monitoring tests in detail, including descriptions of the CD4 cell count and viral load tests.) Labs will also be taken to screen for other infections, such as syphilis, toxoplasmosis, and hepatitis. In addition to these blood tests, you may also be asked to supply a urine sample to check if you are pregnant or have a bladder or pelvic infection. A skin test for tuberculosis may be also done. This sounds like a lot, but these tests will only require urinating into a sterile cup, allowing a nurse to draw a few vials of blood, and having the skin test placed for the tuberculosis screening (which is a quick and tiny pinprick, not a big needle).

Beyond these physical tests, you may also have the opportunity to talk with a nurse and possibly a primary care provider, a social worker, and a health educator. Bring your questions, and do not be embarrassed to share what comes to mind. There are no stupid questions. There are no silly concerns. You should expect to be taken seriously and to be treated with respect. At your first visit, be sure to ask what you should do if you have an urgent problem before your next scheduled visit.

What to Expect at Return Visits

The primary care provider will probably see you at the second visit if she or he did not meet with you at your first visit. The provider generally reviews your medical history, performs a complete physical exam that may include a Pap smear, and discusses your lab results if they are available. He or she will probably discuss whether or not HIV treatments are advisable for you based on your history and laboratory results. If they are, and you decide to start treatment, ask about opportunities to enroll in clinical studies. Your provider should be able to educate you about these options. (Chapter 19 is devoted to the topic of clinical trials and studies.)

Other important concerns that may be discussed at return visits include your general health, reproductive options and birth control, diet, mood, any relationship problems, responses to treatment, applying for disability (if appropriate), managing responsibilities, and any other issues that may be on your mind. You may also be offered specific vaccinations on your first and second visit to protect you from diseases that are of greater concern for people with weakened immune systems. (Chapter 4 discusses these protective vaccinations in greater detail.) Adjusting to healthy life with HIV may require a new open-mindedness toward medical support for many people. The important thing to remember is that close cooperation and good communication with your health care team can keep you well.

How to Have the Most Productive Clinic Visit

• Always bring all of your medications with you. If you are not able to bring all the prescription bottles, then bring a list of what you are actually taking and what doses have been prescribed. This is important, in case your medical chart is not available.
• If you had a medical visit or admission elsewhere, bring the records from that visit if possible. If you cannot easily get the records, be sure to bring the name of the provider who took care of you and the name of the hospital or office.

- Be prepared to wait. Even in the most efficient clinics, people may have long waits. Bring something to keep yourself occupied. Snacks are a good idea.
- If you must leave at a certain time, be sure to let the nurse know about your time limit when you check in.
- Dress comfortably in clothes that you can easily change in and out of.
- Write down a list of questions or topics you want to cover during the visit so you will not forget. This is a very useful habit to develop. Consider keeping a notebook around the house for this purpose, so that you can conveniently jot down your thoughts where they won't be lost between visits.
- Try to arrange to have your labs drawn two weeks before your routine follow-up clinic visit. This way your primary care provider will already know your test results at the time of your visit and will be ready to discuss them with you.
- Check with your primary care provider to find out whether you need to fast before your blood is drawn for any of your lab tests. If so, it is best to schedule an early morning appointment to have the blood drawn so that most of your fasting takes place while you sleep. Simply eat and drink nothing the evening before, get your blood drawn early the next day, and then have breakfast. Many people even bring breakfast with them to avoid further delay.
- Ask your primary care provider for the results of important labs such as your CD4 cell count, viral load, and Pap smear, and keep track of these results. A sample tracking sheet is included in appendix 1 at the end of this book.
- Before each appointment, review your medications to see if you need any refills.
- If you want your prescriptions called in, bring the phone number of your pharmacy.
- If your medications look different when they are refilled, check with your provider before you take them, to make sure they are the correct medications.

Finally, ideally you should develop a close working relationship with your primary care provider over time. Be sure you feel comfortable with your providers and how they interact with you. Do they review all your test results and explain why you need to have the tests performed? Do they let you have input into important decisions such as choosing your HIV treatments? Your primary care provider should be a crucial source of information and should empower you by sharing their expertise and knowledge.

KEY POINTS

1. Ideally, the clinic providing your primary care should offer comprehensive services on site.

2. In the first two clinic visits, expect to have blood drawn, a medical history taken, a physical examination and Pap smear conducted, and your questions answered.

3. Your primary care provider will monitor how you are doing by talking with you, checking for symptoms, looking for physical findings, and following blood test results.

3

HIV, the Immune System, and Monitoring Tests

What is the best way to monitor your HIV infection?

What is the CD4 cell count and viral load?

When do you start having symptoms from your HIV infection?

What is the average time it takes someone to turn from having HIV to having a diagnosis of AIDS?

The human immunodeficiency virus (HIV) hurts the body by attacking its immune system. HIV is a viral infection that weakens a person's ability to fight off other infections of all kinds. Two critical blood tests allow primary care providers to monitor their patients' responses to HIV infection: the absolute CD4 cell count and the viral load. Each of these tests is explained below.

CD4 Cell Count

CD4 cells are also called "T4" or "T-helper" cells. These cells are an important part of the immune system and are a central target of HIV;

therefore, knowing how the CD4 cell count changes over time powerful tool for determining the effect of different treatments. Whe a combination of medicines is working well or when the body is fighting HIV effectively on its own, the CD4 cell count will hold steady or rise. A drop in the CD4 cell count signals a weakening of the body's defenses and suggests that a different treatment approach might be needed. In addition to the absolute *number* of CD4 cells in the body, the *percent* of CD4 cells in the body is also commonly measured. The number fluctuates more than the percent, so if you see a large change in your absolute CD4 cell count, ask your doctor if your CD4 percent also changed. You may be reassured if the percent stays the same, even though the absolute cell count may have appeared to suffer a large drop.

The CD4 cell count (also called the "T-cell count") generally stays above 800 in healthy, HIV-negative adults. While a count of 500 does reveal some minimal damage to the immune system, a person will not develop high risk for infections or complications unless the count drops below 200. Persons are defined as having AIDS if (1) they develop certain health problems because of their damaged immune system, or (2) they have a CD4 cell count less than 200. A person with HIV and a CD4 count above 200 is not defined as having AIDS unless she has developed one of the specific health problems or "AIDS-defining illnesses." Experts generally agree that medical treatment is recommended for anyone with a CD4 count below 200 (these treatments are discussed at length in chapter 6). It is not unusual for a person to see her CD4 count rise with HIV treatment and for the regained cells to work well, protecting against other infections.

Viral Load Tests

The second type of HIV monitoring test measures the "viral load," that is, how much HIV is in the blood. There are two types of viral load tests, but both essentially measure genetic material of the virus. The first test measures branched chain DNA (bDNA). The second is called "quantitative HIV RNA-PCR." The two tests are similar but not iden-

not give the same results, so it may be difficult to track
f two consecutive tests are not of the same kind.
ı person's viral load, the higher her risk of immune sys-
viral load over 100,000 in either test is considered high,
ɔ strict ranges that define "high" or "low" results. Levels greater than one million are possible. The sensitivity of current tests makes it possible to measure viral loads as low as less than 50. In deciding when to recommend treatment for a particular patient, primary care providers consider both the CD4 cell count and the viral load. The goal of treatment is to bring the viral load down to undetectable levels.

How HIV Spreads in the Body

Once HIV has gained access to a person's bloodstream, the envelope surrounding the virus attaches to receptors on the CD4 cells and fuses to the cell surface, allowing the virus to enter. Entry of the virus into cells is helped by "chemokine receptors" named CCR5 and CXCR4. The virus can't infect your cells if the attachment is stopped, the chemokine receptors are blocked, or fusion is inhibited. The first fusion inhibitor, Fuzeon, was recently approved as an HIV treatment. Attachment, chemokine receptors, and fusion inhibitors are called "entry inhibitors." Although the only entry inhibitor on the market today is Fuzeon, several under study may be available in the near future.

Once in the cells, the genetic material of the virus (RNA) undergoes a complicated process called reverse transcription, which means that it is decoded and that its code is used to build new HIV genetic material called HIV-DNA. The enzyme that performs this work is called "reverse transcriptase." This enzyme can be stopped by several available "reverse transcriptase inhibitor" HIV treatments.

The HIV-DNA is next integrated into your chromosomes or the genetic material in your body's cells. The HIV "integrase" is the enzyme essential for accomplishing this task. "Integrase-inhibitors" are another new class of drugs under study that may be available in the future. Once integrated into a cell, the HIV can remain inactive until the cell becomes activated. It is not clear what activates cells or why HIV may suddenly become active.

Once activated, the infected cell's DNA reproduces to make new HIV viruses that emerge from cells back into the bloodstream to seek new host cells to infect. This emergence relies on a different enzyme, called protease, which separates newly reproduced viruses from the host cells. Fortunately, the protease enzyme can be stopped with powerful or potent treatments called "protease inhibitors" that are currently available.

The Effects of HIV Infection
Acute Infection

When HIV gains access to a person's bloodstream, the virus travels to the nearest lymph nodes. Lymph nodes are part of the immune system and are located throughout the body. You may have felt your own lymph nodes swell in your neck when you have had a head cold, for example. They feel like soft lumps and can sometimes be tender. Once inside the nodes, HIV multiplies quickly. The blood then carries the virus to other organs and tissues. For this reason, it is not possible to cure HIV by replacing infected blood with uninfected blood. Blood carries the virus but does not contain it from spreading to other cells. Viral load testing will reveal large amounts of HIV in the blood within a few weeks of initial infection.

At least half of newly infected people will experience some sort of illness during the first one to six weeks. Many will assume they are simply sick with a regular cold virus because the early symptoms of HIV infection resemble those of the common cold. These may include fever, sweats, fatigue, achiness, joint pain, weight loss, headaches, sore throat, swollen lymph nodes, and a general sick feeling. Some people will also have a rash. When a person reports such symptoms to a health care provider, she will likely be tested for mononucleosis, another common infection that shares these symptoms.

The reaction of the body to any infection is to make defensive proteins called antibodies. This takes time—usually about three to twelve weeks. The blood tests that are done to look for HIV are seeking particular antibodies to HIV. If the blood is drawn before many antibodies have been made, the early test result may be negative (see chapter 1). However, the test will turn positive when repeated later after more antibodies have been made. This turning point—when HIV-infected blood yields a positive rather than a falsely negative test result—is the point known as *seroconversion*. At this point antibodies are rallied to fight, and the viral load (the amount of HIV in the blood) rapidly decreases.

Asymptomatic Period

Most people feel good for several years after seroconversion. During this asymptomatic period, a person may not be aware that she is infected with HIV unless she has had an HIV blood test. Indeed, most people with HIV are asymptomatic. Unfortunately, the virus is still active and is reproducing during this symptom-free time, which may last for years. Damage to the immune system can be monitored with tests of the CD4 cell count and of the viral load. Over time, those who do not get effective treatment will usually see a drop in their CD4 cell count and a rise in their viral load. (See figure 3.1.)

Long-term studies of HIV-infected people have found that it typically takes seven to eleven years for an *untreated* person to develop AIDS (although it is important to note that most of these studies have looked at males, not females). Recall that AIDS refers to the complications that arise when the immune system has been significantly damaged by HIV infection, specifically when the CD4 cell count has dropped below 200. These complications are described in chapter 5. A few people have developed AIDS very quickly, only one or two years after initial infection, but this is not typical. On the other hand, 5 to 12 percent of people with HIV infection appear never to progress to AIDS, even without treatment! These people are called *non-progressors*. They likely started out with especially strong immune systems or else they were infected with a weaker strain of HIV. Non-progressors main-

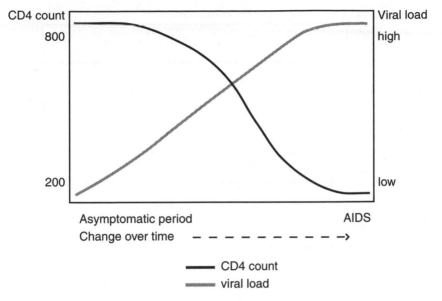

Fig. 3.1. How CD4 Cell Counts and Viral Load Change over Time

tain a high CD4 cell count and a low viral load. Figure 3.2 shows what happens to the CD4 cell count in different populations.

Notice that the non-progressors enjoy a steady and high CD4 count over time. *Untreated* progressors have a drop in the CD4 count over time. But *treated* progressors see the initial drop in CD4 cells reverse when treatment begins, and the CD4 count returns to a high level. A summary of what happens to the CD4 cell count and viral load levels in untreated persons is shown in table 3.1.

The Progression from HIV Infection to AIDS

Current HIV treatments can greatly extend the length of the asymptomatic period, possibly for the infected person's entire lifetime. This is remarkable progress since the early days of the epidemic when virtually no treatment was available and when outcomes were very poor. Now, people with HIV can feel well.

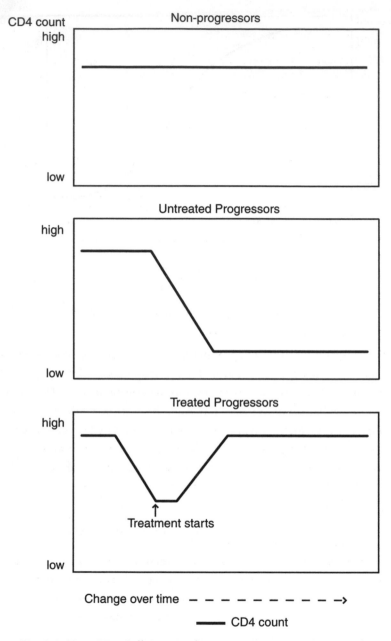

Fig. 3.2. How CD4 Cell Counts Change in Non-progressors, People Receiving Treatment, and People Not Receiving Treatment

Table 3.1
Review of CD4 Cell Count and Viral Load Changes in Untreated People

1. During acute infection, the viral load is very high. The CD4 cell count is also generally high, since the virus has not yet had the opportunity to undermine the immune system.
2. As the immune system makes antibodies to fight HIV, the HIV test will turn positive and the viral load will start to drop to very low levels.
3. During the asymptomatic period, the viral load may stay very low for a long time or may slowly start to rise. As the viral load rises, the CD4 cell count falls.
4. HIV-related symptoms increase as the viral load increases and as the CD4 cell count decreases.
5. A person with HIV has AIDS only when blood tests show a CD4 cell count below 200 or when the person develops specific health problems related to their damaged immune system.

Primary care providers should discuss HIV treatment options with any patients whose CD4 cell counts and viral load test results meet certain levels, as explained in chapter 6. Factors that may influence the length of the asymptomatic period include the strain of HIV circulating in the blood (since some strains are weaker than others) and the strength of the person's immune system before infection. This last factor can be related to age. For example, very young and very old populations are less resilient than people at other ages. It is not known whether other factors such as stress, recreational drug use, pre-existing medical conditions, or diet play an important role in determining the length of the asymptomatic period.

Although most of the studies of HIV's progression to AIDS have been based on men, their results seem to apply to women, as well. This has become increasingly clear in recent years. Early on in the epidemic, women were not considered a population at high risk for HIV, so by the time many ill women were even tested for HIV, they had already progressed to AIDS. This delay in medical care meant that little research could be done on women with HIV who had not progressed to AIDS.

Today, however, women are fully recognized as a population at risk for HIV and are therefore referred for testing and treatment much earlier in the course of the disease. Chapter 4 explores the progression from HIV infection to AIDS in greater detail.

Today we know that women with HIV do not get sick from the infection any faster than men do. However, there are some sex differences. If you compare infected women and men who have the same high CD4 cell count, women will have lower viral loads than the men—that is, the women will have a lower concentration of HIV in their blood. At lower CD4 counts, however, this difference is not seen. *These interesting observations may lead health care providers to suggest starting HIV treatments for women at lower viral load levels than the guidelines discussed in chapter 6.* Some believe the observed difference is related to hormones. While pregnancy does not appear to influence the progression from HIV to AIDS, little is known about the possible effects on progression of hormone treatments such as birth control pills or hormone replacement therapy.

What can an infected person do to stay as healthy as possible for as long as possible? Here are some guidelines:

- Eat a well-balanced, nutritional diet. You may wish to consult a dietitian for advice about what to eat.
- Avoid harm to your body through smoking, alcohol, drugs, and excessive caffeine.
- Try to avoid stress in your life.
- Start or continue an exercise program you enjoy.
- Keep appointments with your primary care provider and follow their advice on any recommendations or treatments that prevent illness and HIV-related complications.
- Monitor what is happening in your body by having your CD4 cell count and viral load checked (usually every three months). Your primary care provider will discuss HIV treatment options when blood tests show that treatment may be beneficial. (See chapter 6 for a discussion on when to start treatment.)

KEY POINTS

1. *The CD4 cell count is a test used to monitor the effect of HIV infection on the immune system. At counts near and below 200, the body becomes susceptible to certain infections that previously had been easier to fight off.*

2. *Viral load testing measures how much HIV is in the blood, which depends on how active the virus is. An infection is very active if viral loads exceed 100,000. HIV treatments can often decrease viral loads to levels so low they cannot be detected by current tests.*

3. *Many people newly infected with HIV will have viral symptoms. The HIV screening test may not be positive until three months after a person becomes infected.*

4. *Most people infected with HIV have no symptoms for several years.*

5. *Seven to eleven years usually pass before an untreated person with HIV develops AIDS.*

PART TWO

Meeting the Challenge
of HIV Infection

HIV is a powerful virus. For people infected with the virus who do not receive treatment, the virus can cause many complications. By weakening the body's immune system, HIV makes a person vulnerable to infections and diseases. In the past, before HIV was well understood, the medical system could do very little to help people with HIV avoid these other infections. Today, however, things are different. We know much more about the immune system and about this disease than ever before. We can detect problems earlier and with greater accuracy. We have stronger and more targeted medications. We have health care providers expertly trained to manage HIV. We have excellent HIV clinics equipped with many services and specialty doctors. And we are conducting ongoing studies and clinical trials to increase our understanding of HIV and to increase the effectiveness of medical treatment.

4

Recognizing Symptoms and
Preventing Complications

---

*What are the symptoms and complications of
HIV infection?*

What is AIDS? Is it the same thing as HIV?

How can HIV-related complications be prevented?

Not everyone with HIV is sick. In fact, most people have no symptoms
at all right after they are infected with HIV. However, after a few years
the virus destroys parts of the immune system and makes it more difficult for the body to defend against other infections. As described in
chapter 3, the amount of immune system damage caused by the HIV is
monitored by a blood test called the CD4 cell count (also called the "T-
cell count"). HIV-related symptoms generally occur when the CD4 cell
count is low, particularly if it falls below 200.

In the past, before strong HIV treatments were available, the complications described in this chapter were common in people with HIV.
Things are different now. Preventing complications is the name of the
game. While it is important to understand the complications that may
possibly occur, it is equally important to understand that HIV treat-

ments can help prevent these complications. This chapter can serve as a guide to complications if you ever need it.

First HIV-Related Symptoms

In women, one of the first symptoms of HIV infection is often a vaginal yeast infection that keeps coming back. The medical term for vaginal yeast is *Candida vaginitis* or *vulvovaginal Candidiasis*. In one study, nearly 40 percent of women with HIV visited a health care provider because they had a vaginal yeast infection. Other gynecological problems that are common among women with HIV are abnormal Pap smears, genital warts, pelvic infections, and vaginal sores. Many women without HIV develop these conditions, but if you don't know whether you have HIV and you do have one of these conditions, you should consider getting tested for HIV. Note that gynecologic infections and other sexually transmitted diseases are discussed in detail in chapter 8.

Nongynecologic symptoms are generally the same for both men and women with HIV. There are some exceptions: more women with HIV than men with HIV are anemic (that is, they have a lower than normal red blood count), and women with HIV tend to have more frequent thrush (oral candidiasis) and serious bacterial infections (such as pneumonia) than men do. Common nongynecologic symptoms are described below in alphabetical order.

Nongynecologic HIV-Related Symptoms
Anemia (Low Red Blood Cell Count)

Many women, even those without HIV, have anemia. It often results from a lack of iron, which the body needs to make blood. Women who are menstruating lose blood with each period. The body's need for iron also increases during pregnancy. Iron-deficiency anemia can be treated with iron supplements or with a diet rich in iron. Such a diet would include meat and green leafy vegetables. Iron-enriched cereals are another good source of iron.

In addition to iron deficiency, certain medical conditions, such as HIV-infection, can lower the blood count. Some HIV treatments, particularly Retrovir (zidovudine or AZT), can also cause anemia. Your primary care provider can usually determine the cause of your anemia with blood tests.

A woman may not realize that she is anemic until her blood count is checked. Some women simply have no symptoms. Some, on the other hand, may feel fatigued, weak, dizzy, or just lacking their usual energy. Iron supplements can treat iron-deficiency anemia but will not help with other types of anemia. For these, different medicines are prescribed that stimulate the bone to produce more red blood cells—for example, the drugs Procrit and Epogen (erythropoietin). These medicines are usually successful in treating anemia caused by HIV or HIV treatments; someone with an iron deficiency will still need to take iron supplements. Unfortunately Procrit and Epogen must be injected underneath the skin about once a week. If you feel bad and your blood count is very low, your primary care provider may also recommend that you receive a red blood cell transfusion.

Bacterial Pneumonia

Bacterial pneumonia is a lung infection. It causes fever, shortness of breath, and cough. Pneumonia can be serious and may require hospitalization. It is more common among smokers and those who use injectable street drugs. To treat pneumonia, antibiotics are either taken by mouth or administered through an IV line inserted into a vein. Different bacteria can cause pneumonia. The bacteria that most often cause pneumonia are *Streptococcus pneumoniae* or just "pneumococcus." Although there is now a vaccine for this bacteria, the vaccine does not contain every existing strain of pneumococcus, and not all patients' immune systems respond completely to the vaccine. Therefore, the vaccine can offer some protection against pneumococcal infections, but it is not 100 percent effective. It also does not protect against pneumonias caused by other, non-streptococcal infections, such as *Pneumocystis carinii* pneumonia (described later in this chapter).

Diarrhea

Some medicines cause diarrhea as a side effect. Both antibiotics and some HIV treatments (such as Viracept and Kaletra) cause diarrhea in many people. Certain HIV-related infections with viruses, bacteria, or parasites (such as *Mycobacterium avium-intracellulare*, cryptosporidiosis, and microsporidiosis) can also cause diarrhea. These infections are diagnosed by culturing the organism from the stool or by looking at a stool sample under a microscope. The treatment for diarrhea depends on the cause. Imodium or Lomotil can help to slow down the diarrhea, and calcium supplements often control diarrhea caused by Viracept.

Fatigue (Lack of Energy)

Fatigue is very common even among HIV-negative women. Without adequate relaxation, exercise, and time for self-nurture, people feel fatigued. Stress and worries can also interfere with sleep and leave us feeling drained of energy. Working to achieve regular sleep and a nutritious diet will help, as will daily multivitamins. But medical reasons for fatigue, such as anemia or depression, require different treatments. When HIV infection is the cause of fatigue, starting HIV treatments will often increase energy and bring a heightened sense of well-being.

Lymphadenopathy (Swollen Lymph Nodes)

Swollen lymph nodes or "knots" can occur around the neck, under the arms, and in the groin area. When they are due to HIV infection, swollen lymph nodes are generally not painful. These nodes do *not* mean that the HIV infection is progressing. Sometimes lymph nodes swell in response to other infections or (rarely) to cancer, but usually these causes bring additional symptoms such as fever and weight loss. Lymph nodes also sometimes swell after a person starts HIV treatments for the first time, probably because the immune system is responding so well.

If there is concern about what is causing the lymph nodes to swell, taking a biopsy of the lymph node may reveal the cause. A biopsy is taken by sticking a needle into the node, drawing out some of the tissue, and examining it under a microscope. When lymphadenopathy is caused by cancer or by infection other than HIV, the underlying cause of the swollen nodes usually needs to be treated. No treatment is necessary for lymphadenopathy associated only with HIV infection.

Myalgia (Muscle Pain) and Neuropathy (Nerve Pain)

HIV can cause general achiness in the muscles (myalgia) and discomfort in the nerves (neuropathy). In addition to HIV, another cause of myalgia is inflamed muscles, which can be a side effect from some HIV treatments or medications used to treat abnormal blood fat levels (such as high cholesterol levels). If you have sore muscles, your primary care provider may want to check specific blood tests. Generally nonsteroidal anti-inflammatory drugs (NSAIDs) such as Advil and Aleve are used to treat myalgia.

Most people describe the discomfort of neuropathy as numbness, tingling, or pain in the feet, legs, fingers, or hands. This discomfort might come and go, or it may persist. Certain medications, such as some of the HIV treatments discussed in chapter 6, can cause neuropathy or make it worse. The diagnosis of neuropathy is usually based on a description of symptoms rather than on any medical testing. Yet sometimes blood tests can identify vitamin deficiencies or diseases like diabetes, which can also cause neuropathy. When HIV treatments are thought to be causing the neuropathy, changing the treatment regimen may help. There are also pain medications for this condition, such as Neurontin (gabapentin), Elavil (amitriptyline), and opioid therapies. (Chapter 17 discusses pain management at length.)

Oral Candidiasis (Thrush)

Thrush is a painful but usually easy-to-treat yeast infection of the mouth. It can extend down the esophagus (the tube connecting the mouth to the stomach) as well. Thrush looks like cottage cheese. It can cause difficulty eating and swallowing. Fortunately, a course of one of the following medications will usually clear the infection. The topical treatments, Nystatin swish and swallow or Mycelex (clotrimazole) troches that are sucked, are usually the first medications tried. Using the topical treatments first is preferable because thrush tends to become resistant to oral treatments over time if a person chronically stays on them.

If the topical treatments do not work, Diflucan (fluconazol) pills generally work well. Patients who have developed resistance to Diflucan may still be sensitive to Sporonox (itraconazole) swish and swallow. Additional treatments that can be tried include fungizone (oral amphoterin) swish and swallow or Vfend (voriconazole) pills. You should not take Vfend if you are pregnant. If oral and topical medications fail to work, then amphotericin can be given through an IV, directly into a vein.

Rashes

Several annoying and sometimes serious rashes can accompany HIV infection. One rash, called *seborrheic dermatitis*, most often occurs on the face, causing dry, flaky skin around the nose and between the eyebrows. It can be treated with topical steroid or anti-fungal creams. Another rash, called *eosinophilic folliculitis*, causes itchy bumps over the body. It may respond to a light treatment known as phototherapy, which can be done in an outpatient office. Benadryl, taken by mouth, can decrease the itching but may cause drowsiness.

Herpes zoster, or shingles, is a very uncomfortable and sometimes painful rash caused by the chicken pox virus. It is a relatively common rash among persons with HIV, especially those with low CD4 cell counts. Once someone has chicken pox, the chicken pox virus never leaves the body, and the rash can emerge years or even decades after the initial chicken pox infection. The rash is usually located on only one area of the body, and its small blisters resemble chicken pox. It is not serious unless it covers the whole body or affects the eyes or lungs or brain. Several treatments can shorten the time of the rash, but none will cure it. The rash of herpes zoster often comes back again. Treatments include Zovirax (acyclovir), Famvir (famciclovir), and Valtrex (valacyclovir). Usually pain medication is also required. (See chapter 17 for a discussion on how to treat nerve pain.

Kaposi's sarcoma (described below), one of the AIDS-defining illnesses, is a type of cancer that causes purple and red skin bumps. It is very uncommon among women. If a primary care provider thinks a rash might be Kaposi's sarcoma, she or he will recommend a skin biopsy to find out. Rarely will any of the other rashes described need a biopsy, since they can generally be diagnosed with confidence by how they look.

Weight Loss

There are many causes of weight loss. Decreased appetite, nausea, vomiting, diarrhea, or difficulty chewing or swallowing can all potentially lead to weight loss. People may also lose weight or have trouble putting on weight just from HIV infection. Your primary care provider should try to determine the cause of any weight loss so that treatment can be targeted. For example, if a patient is losing weight because she has a treatable mouth infection like thrush that makes eating painful, then treating the thrush should halt the weight loss. In addition to taking treatments for the possible causes of weight loss, people with HIV can add calorie-rich nutritional supplements such as Ensure to their diets to gain weight. If you are able to get your HIV infection under control by taking HIV treatments, you may gain back any weight you lost.

Medical therapies to improve the appetite include Megace (megestrol acetate), Serostim (human growth hormone), Marinol (dronabinol), and anabolic treatments such as Anadrol (oxymetholone) or Oxandrin (oxandrolone). Megace (megestrol acetate), a progesterone agent, causes fat weight gain, and the anabolic therapies cause muscle weight gain. The anabolic agents are related to testosterone, a male sex hormone. Anadrol and Oxadrin have been shown to be safe in women, though they can cause certain side effects such as deepening of the voice, changes in sex drive, abnormal hair growth, and acne. All of the hormonal therapies (Megace, anabolic agents) can affect a woman's menstrual periods. Serostim has to be injected and is very expensive, costing at least $12,000 for a course of treatment. Marinol, a derivative of marijuana, also helps control nausea.

The Difference between HIV Infection and AIDS

If an HIV-infected person has a CD4 cell count below 200 or one or more of the atypical medical conditions described in the next section, she is diagnosed with AIDS—Acquired Immune Deficiency Syndrome. If her CD4 cell count is over 200 and she does not have one of the specified medical conditions, she is diagnosed with HIV infection but not with AIDS. The medical conditions described in the next section are called "AIDS-defining opportunistic processes." They include specific infections, cancers, and syndromes. While the following section lists many AIDS-defining processes and conditions, it is important to remember that *not all people with AIDS experience all of these conditions.*

AIDS-Defining Opportunistic Processes or Conditions

There are more than twenty AIDS-defining medical conditions among adults. The most frequent conditions among both women and men are *Pneumocystis carinii* pneumonia (PCP), *Candida* esophagitis, and "wasting syndrome," which means the loss of at least 10 percent of body weight. Recommendations for preventing some of these conditions are discussed at the end of this chapter.

The more frequent opportunistic processes are described below, in alphabetical order. Other AIDS-defining diagnoses discussed elsewhere in this book include wasting syndrome, recurrent bacterial pneumonia, invasive cervical cancer (see chapter 9), and chronic genital sores caused by herpes simplex virus (see chapter 8).

Candida Esophagitis (Thrush)

As mentioned above, thrush is more frequent among women than men. If thrush is in the mouth, it can spread down into the esophagus (the tube connecting the mouth to the stomach). This may cause both difficulty swallowing and chest pain. Some people report the feeling that something is "stuck" in their chests. Diflucan (fluconazole) is a pill that can treat this infection. If Diflucan does not work well, Vfend (voriconazole) may be another option. If both of these medications fail to control the problem, then a procedure called endoscopy is usually recommended. An endoscope is a tube with a light that a specialist gently guides down the esophagus so that it can be clearly visualized. If anything looks abnormal, the doctor can take a tissue sample to determine whether or not persistent symptoms are due to a *Candida* infection.

Cryptococcal Meningitis

Cryptococcus neoformans is a fungus that often goes to the brain, where it can infect the lining around the spinal cord and brain. This condition is known as meningitis. *Cryptococcus* is an inhaled fungus that can also infect the bloodstream or cause pneumonia. If you have cryptococcal meningitis, you probably will have a headache and fever. This infection is diagnosed by looking at the cerebrospinal fluid (CSF) that surrounds the brain. The CSF is obtained through a procedure called a spinal tap. A spinal tap is done by sticking a needle through a hole between two bones in the spinal column to draw out the cerebrospinal fluid. This test is relatively safe and can be done in clinic. If you have a spinal tap, you will be advised to lie down for an hour after the test to decrease the chances of developing a headache.

Once begun, treatment for cryptococcal meningitis is generally not stopped but is continued for life. The medications that treat *Cryptococcus* are Diflucan (by mouth or vein) or amphotericin (only through the vein). Some limited studies have suggested that Vfend (voriconazole) may also work for those who do not respond to Diflucan. If treatment is stopped, cryptococcal meningitis is very likely to come back. However, a few people who greatly improved their immune systems after starting HIV treatments have been reported to do well after stopping their cryptococcal treatment. The U.S. Public Health Service and Infectious Disease Society of America recommends that therapy may be stopped after the initial course of treatment in people without symptoms who have maintained CD4 cell counts greater than 100 to 200 for at least six months.

Cryptosporidiosis

Cryptosporidium is a parasite that contaminates drinking water. To avoid infection with cryptosporidiosis, anyone with HIV, particularly those with immune system damage, should either boil their drinking water or drink only bottled water. Ideally, any contact with human or animal stools should also be avoided (for example, changing diapers and changing litter boxes). Pets, especially those younger than six months, can be infected with cryptosporidiosis. If you plan to get a new pet, you should have the animal's stools checked. You do not need to give away healthy pets you already own.

If you have cryptosporidiosis, you may experience diarrhea and frequent stools. While there is no good medical treatment for cryptosporidiosis, some people are able to clear the infection on their own. One possible way to cure the infection is to improve your immune system through HIV treatment. Medications to control the diarrhea can also help relieve symptoms.

Cytomegalovirus Infection

Many adults have been infected with the virus called cytomegalovirus (CMV). It is both common and contagious. CMV is often transmitted in day-care settings, and people often catch the infection from their children. Good hand washing decreases the risk of catching the infection. CMV can also be transmitted through sex, but condoms protect against infection.

Just because a person has been infected with CMV does not mean that the virus remains active. Many people carry CMV without knowing it. However, for people with HIV whose CD4 cell counts drop below 50, CMV may be difficult to keep under control. When active, CMV can cause retinitis, an inflammation of the back of the eye. Untreated CMV retinitis is serious and can lead to blindness. To catch the infection early, it is a good idea to have an experienced provider (usually an ophthalmologist) check the back of your eyes every three months if your CD4 cell count is less than 100. Rarely, CMV can also infect the gastrointestinal tract and cause bloody diarrhea and stomach pain. Sometimes it can also infect the brain, causing confusion, weakness, and even paralysis.

Although CMV cannot be cured, it can usually be controlled by medications, including Cytovene (ganciclovir), Vistide (cidofovir), Foscavir (foscarnet), and Valcyte (valganciclovir). With the exception of Valcyte and Cytovene, these medications are given through the vein. Cytovene by mouth is not strong enough to be given by itself when a person is first diagnosed with CMV, but it can also be delivered to the eye through shots or implants that are changed every six months. The implants are placed in a hospital setting, but an overnight stay is not necessary. People generally stay on anti-CMV treatment for the rest of their lives, but if HIV treatments are effective in raising a person's CD4 cell count and keeping it above the 100–150 range, anti-CMV therapy might reasonably be stopped.

HIV-Related Encephalitis/Dementia

HIV infection can cause problems with memory and concentration, especially in people over the age of 40. Yet when people report these symptoms, it is always important to look for other possible causes. Imaging studies of the head, such as computerized tomography (CT) and magnetic resonance imaging (MRI) scans, and blood tests can help identify the source of the symptoms. CT and MRI scans are painless, noninvasive procedures that allow health care providers to see details of organs and tissue inside the body. The machines are high-tech cameras. To have one of these scans done, you lie down on a flat table inside a long, tubular machine while it takes a series of pictures of your head. The resulting images can reveal brain inflammation (encephalitis) as well as any fluid collections or solid tissue that might be creating pressure on the brain and causing symptoms. Unfortunately, there is no specific treatment for HIV encephalitis, but symptoms are likely to improve with HIV treatment.

Kaposi's Sarcoma

Kaposi's sarcoma is rare in women. Unlike men, women with Kaposi's sarcoma are more likely to have this cancer spread to internal organs, particularly the lungs. If the cancer is limited to the skin, it is treated with radiation therapy or injected with anti-tumor drugs. If it has spread, chemotherapy is generally recommended.

Mycobacterium avium Complex Infections

Mycobacterium avium complex (MAC) is a bacterium related to tuberculosis, but it is not contagious and its symptoms are usually not as severe. It is usually diagnosed with a blood culture. MAC blood infection may bring high fevers, weight loss, diarrhea, cough, and a general feeling of sickness. To prevent infection with MAC, people with CD4 cell counts below 50 are advised to take prophylactic antibiotics.

The easiest preventative antibiotic to take is Zithromax (azithromycin), since it only requires taking two pills once each week. Biaxin (clarithromycin) and Mycobutin (rifabutin) also work against MAC but require more frequent dosing. Prevention with antibiotics is important, because this infection is difficult to control. It responds poorly to drug treatment. Therefore, people with a MAC blood infection generally stay on two to five antibiotics for life or until HIV treatments raise the CD4 cell count above the vulnerable range. Mycobutin interacts with several HIV treatments, so dosages of medications often have to be adjusted. The U.S. Public Health Service and Infectious Disease Society of America has recommended that therapy can be discontinued in persons who have received at least twelve months of treatment, have no symptoms due to MAC, and have had a CD4 cell count over 100 for at least six months.

Pneumocystis carinii Pneumonia

Pneumocystis carinii pneumonia (PCP) is a serious fungal infection that threatens the immune system when the CD4 cell count drops below 200. To prevent PCP, persons with HIV should take protective medicines if their CD4 counts are less than 200 or if they have thrush. Effective medications include Bactrim (trimethoprim-sulfamethoxazole), dapsone, Mepron (atovaquone), and Pentam (pentamidine).

PCP infection may cause fever, shortness of breath, and cough. It is usually suspected, based on these findings, and then diagnosed with the combination of a chest X-ray and a test for the level of oxygen in the blood. Sometimes a bronchoscopy is required to confirm the diagnosis. A bronchoscope is a lighted tube gently guided through the mouth, down the trachea, and into the lungs, allowing for retrieval of lung secretions that can then be definitively tested for the presence of fungus.

If caught early, PCP can be treated outside of the hospital. However, PCP can become life-threatening if treatment is delayed. Fortunately, the treatment takes only three weeks and is considered curative.

Toxoplasma Encephalitis

Toxoplasma gondii is a parasite that can grow in the brain, creating bundles of infection called abscesses. People with HIV who have been exposed to this parasite become vulnerable to toxoplasmosis when CD4 counts drop below 100. Preventative antibiotics such as Bactrim (trimethoprim-sulfamethoxazole), Mepron (atovaquone), or Daraprim (pyrimethamine) are always recommended for persons with a CD4 cell count less than 100 and positive antibodies (determined by a blood test) for toxoplasmosis. If the CD4 cell count increases to greater than 200 for at least three months, the preventive antibiotics can be stopped.

Toxoplasmosis can also infect cats, but there are no recommendations to test cats for the infection or to avoid cats. The parasite lives in the stool of infected cats, so no one with HIV should touch cat stools, which can be unintentionally encountered when gardening. Gloves are always recommended when working in the soil. If it is necessary to manage a litter box, then careful hand washing is very important.

Food can also become contaminated with toxoplasmosis. All fruits and vegetables must be carefully washed. Raw or undercooked meat can also contain toxoplasmosis and should therefore be avoided. These precautions are particularly important if you are pregnant and have never been infected with toxoplasmosis, since a new infection can affect the unborn baby.

Toxoplasmosis can cause weakness in one or more limbs as well as seizures or convulsions. It is diagnosed with either a CT or MRI scan of the head. While the presence of an abscess on either the CT or MRI suggests toxoplasmosis infection, it is still possible that other, less common diagnoses could be the cause. However, toxoplasmosis is the most likely explanation. For this reason, treatment directed against toxoplasmosis is usually started first (either Daraprim plus sulfadiazine or Daraprim plus clindamycin). The CT scan or MRI is then repeated two to three weeks later. If the abscess has not improved, a brain biopsy might be necessary: only a brain biopsy can give the definite diagnosis. Since toxoplasmosis recurs, treatment is generally for life. However, the U.S. Public Health Service and Infectious Disease Society of America recommends that treatment may be stopped after the initial course in people without symptoms who have a CD4 cell count greater than 200 for at least six months.

Tuberculosis

In the 1800s, tuberculosis was a very common disease in America. Known as "consumption," the disease was even believed to run in families because it was so contagious that whole households would come down with it, from grandparents to babies. Unlike today, there was no effective medication for it.

All people who test positive for HIV should be tested for exposure to tuberculosis, a bacterial infection. This test involves a simple skin study called a PPD. A small amount of material is injected just below the surface of the skin. If the skin responds with an area of swelling or a bump (also called induration), the test shows that the person has been exposed to tuberculosis at some time in the past. Having the skin turn pink without swelling does not indicate a positive reaction. *People with very low CD4 cell counts may not show any reaction, even if they have been exposed.* This lack of response even in the presence of prior exposure is called "anergy."

Sometimes people who are infected with tuberculosis will have active and contagious lung infection—pneumonia—and sometimes they will not. A chest X-ray will reveal the presence or absence of pneumonia and is an important follow-up study for anyone with a positive PPD. Pregnant women should *never* have an X-ray without first shielding the abdomen with the lead apron provided by the X-ray technician. X-rays can cause severe deformities in unborn babies. Once a person has shown a positive PPD reaction, his or her skin will always test positive for exposure to tuberculosis, so there is no need to repeat the test. In fact, PPD-positive people can have severe skin reactions to repeat testing.

Anyone who tests positive for tuberculosis exposure needs to be treated. Even if the tuberculosis is silent in the body, causing no sickness, medications are still necessary to keep the disease from becoming active and spreading. When tuberculosis is active, it usually causes a high fever, weight loss, cough (sometimes bloody cough), and shortness of breath. Anyone with a positive HIV test and *active* tubercular pneumonia is diagnosed as having AIDS, but a positive PPD alone does not lead to this diagnosis.

People with active tuberculosis are considered extremely contagious until they have received at least two weeks of treatment. Hospitalization is often recommended for this two-week period. After the first two weeks, medicines can usually be taken outside the hospital.

Treatment for active tuberculosis takes *at least six months*. Several different medicines are given in combination to treat active tuberculosis, and their doses can be raised so that the medicines only need to be taken twice a week. HIV treatments can interact with tuberculosis treatments, requiring dose adjustments in the HIV medications and sometimes limiting HIV treatment options. Two to nine months of treatment is recommended for people with a positive PPD, depending on their medication regimen.

Preventing Complications

Adjusting to life with HIV means adjusting to life with pills. The pills, however, mean that you do not have to adjust to life with terrible sickness. Most people have taken antibiotics at some time or another in their lives, perhaps to treat an ear infection or strep throat. In the last century, these miraculous medications transformed many fatal diseases into diseases we now consider almost trivial. Few parents get terribly worried when their children develop fevers with their head colds. We have whole aisles of pain-relieving and fever-reducing medications, cough-suppressants, decongestants, and more. But most reassuringly, we have antibiotics and antifungals for those times when we need help fighting infection.

HIV is an infection that weakens a person's ability to fight other infections, and therefore antibiotic help is needed more regularly. Taking preventive medicines *before* an infection strikes is called *prophylaxis* and is a powerful means of avoiding serious illness. Table 4.1 lists the antibiotics used to prevent or treat specific conditions. Most antibiotics are safe during pregnancy, but Mepron, PZA, Daraprim, and Biaxin generally should not be taken during pregnancy. The antifungal medication called Diflucan (or fluconazol) generally should not be taken in early pregnancy because of concern about its effects on unborn babies. Pregnant women who need antifungal medication to treat yeast infections like thrush or vaginitis should first use topical treatments and should only turn to the oral Diflucan if these topical treatments fail to work.

Table 4.1
Antibiotics Used to Prevent Important Infections

Condition	Indication	Preferred treatment	Alternative treatment(s)
Pneumocystis carinii pneumonia (PCP)	CD4 less than 200 or presence of thrush	Bactrim	Dapsone* Aerosol Pentam Mepron** Rifadin***
Tuberculosis	Positive TB skin test	Isoniazide (INH) + vitamin B6, or Rifadin + Pyrazinamide (PZA)**	
Toxoplasmosis	Positive antibody test and CD4 less than 100	Bactrim	Daraprim** Mepron**
Mycobacterium avium complex (MAC)	CD4 less than 50	Zithromax Biaxin**	Mycobutin

Note: Bactrim = trimethoprim-sulfamethoxazole; Pentam = pentamidine; Mepron = atovaquone; Rifadin = rifampin; Daraprim = pyrimethamine; Zithromax = azithromycin; Biaxin = clarithromycin; Mycobutin = rifabutin.
* If you have a deficiency of a certain enzyme (G6PD), you should not take dapsone because you may become very anemic.
** Mepron, PZA, Daraprim, and Biaxin should be avoided during pregnancy.
***Mycobutin may be substituted for Rifadin.

In addition to taking HIV medications and prophylactic antibiotics, people with HIV can take vaccinations to prevent some complications. Vaccines stimulate the immune system to produce antibodies against specific infections. People with high CD4 counts have better protective responses to vaccines than people with low counts. This is another reason to take HIV medications: they can raise CD4 cell counts high enough to allow the person to benefit from vaccines. Because vaccines

Table 4.2

Vaccine Recommendations

Condition	Indication	Number of doses
Streptococcus pneumoniae	CD4 greater than 200	1 dose
Hepatitis A	*	2 doses
Hepatitis B	no antibodies**	3 doses
Influenza	all patients	1 dose every fall
Varicella zoster (chicken pox)	exposed and no antibodies*	antibodies (immune globulin) given within 96 hours of exposure

Note: At this time there is no vaccination for hepatitis C.

* Hepatitis A vaccine should be strongly considered by anyone who lacks prior immunity, who has other liver problems such as hepatitis B or C infection, or who has any of the hepatitis A risk factors described in chapter 5.

** See chapter 5 for an explanation of antibodies.

can temporarily increase viral load a bit, more accurate and useful test results will be obtained if you have your viral load test drawn just before you receive the vaccine or not until at least two weeks after vaccination.

If you are pregnant, your obstetrician will probably postpone giving certain vaccinations until after your baby is born so that the baby will not be exposed to the slightly higher viral load that the vaccine might cause. Ideally pregnant women should only receive vaccinations if their viral loads are suppressed to very low levels. However, the influenza vaccine is one that may be particularly important to take during pregnancy (depending on the time of year), and it is generally given when it becomes available in the fall, regardless of viral load level. Table 4.2 lists the vaccinations available for specific conditions.

People who take HIV treatments greatly reduce their chances of developing complications from HIV. All the infections associated with AIDS are avoided when the immune system maintains strength and the CD4 cell count stays high. In fact, many of the infection-preventing treatments like antibiotics can even be stopped if HIV medications boost the immune system to a point where the body can protect itself. See chapter 6 for a discussion of HIV treatments.

KEY POINTS

1. HIV can cause gynecologic symptoms such as vaginal yeast infections, abnormal Pap smears, genital warts, pelvic infections, and vaginal sores.

2. Some conditions, such as anemia (low red blood count), thrush, and bacterial infections, are more common in women than men. Otherwise, women and men have the same HIV-related nongynecologic complaints.

3. HIV-related symptoms are more common in the presence of immune system damage.

4. A diagnosis of AIDS applies only when the CD4 cell count is less than 200 (showing immune system damage) or when one of the specific AIDS-defining infections, cancers, or medical conditions described in this chapter appears.

5. HIV treatments offer the best possible protection against HIV-related complications because they strengthen the immune system. In addition, specific antibiotics and vaccinations protect against infections that may develop when CD4 cell counts are low.

Resources

1. CancerNet at cancernet.nci.nih.gov/Cancer_Types/AIDS-Related_Malignancies.html (information on Kaposi's sarcoma and lymphoma)
2. OncoLink at oncolink.upenn.edu/disease/kaposi/ (information on Kaposi's sarcoma and lymphoma)
3. HIV and Hepatitis.com at www.hivandhepatitis.com (information on hepatitis A, B, and C)
4. CDC, Viral Hepatitis at www.cdc.gov/ncidod/diseases/hepatitis/ (information on hepatitis)

5

Hepatitis and the Liver

What is hepatitis and how is it recognized?

What can you do to protect your liver?

How are hepatitis A, B, and C transmitted?

What are the complications from a chronic hepatitis infection?

How is hepatitis treated?

What Is Hepatitis?

Your liver is a large and important organ. About the size of a football, it sits in the upper part of your abdomen on the right, protected by your rib cage, just below your right lung. The healthy liver does many jobs for the body. It filters toxins; stores and processes sugars; metabolizes fats, carbohydrates, and drugs; and makes blood components and bile. If the liver becomes inflamed, it gets tender and sore.

Hepatitis is an inflammatory disease of the liver. It can be caused by viral infections, certain medications, or excessive alcohol consumption. The most common viral causes of hepatitis are simply called hepatitis A (HAV), hepatitis B (HBV), and hepatitis C (HCV). Other viruses that cause hepatitis are rare, so we will focus only on these three. Although each hepatitis virus can cause acute, severe liver inflammation, only HBV and HCV cause chronic liver problems.

Acute hepatitis causes liver pain, nausea, vomiting, and a general sense of sickness. Another important symptom of liver disease is "jaundice," which refers to a yellowing of the white areas of the eyes. Urine may also turn a bright yellow-orange color. These color changes are due to an excessive buildup of bilirubin in the body. Bilirubin is a natural substance resulting from the normal turnover of red blood cells. It is metabolized by the healthy liver, but if the liver becomes inflamed and stops working well, then bilirubin accumulates. The resulting jaundice also causes general itching. Chronic liver problems that can result from HBV or HCV infection include liver failure, liver cancer, and cirrhosis (an irreversible scarring of the liver).

How You Can Protect Your Liver

If you have hepatitis from any cause, there are things you can do to prevent liver damage. These recommendations are listed below. First of all, you should avoid alcohol, which acts as a poison to the liver. Certain medications can also be toxic to the liver, especially high doses of Tylenol, aspirin, or non-steroidal anti-inflammatory drugs (NSAIDs) like Motrin, Aleve, and Advil. Lower doses of Tylenol (for example less than 500 to 2,000 mg a day) are probably safe, but you should check with your primary care provider before taking any NSAIDs. If you have moderate to severe chronic pain and active hepatitis, the safest type of pain medications are pure opiates (see chapter 17). If blood tests show that you have severe liver inflammation, your provider may even recommend that you stop taking all or most of your medications, even your HIV treatments, for a short period of time until the inflammation subsides.

Fortunately, there are safe and effective vaccines against hepatitis A and B. Both require more than one shot because the body will not produce antibodies at the first vaccine exposure. Hepatitis A vaccine requires two shots separated from each other by six months. Hepatitis B vaccine involves a series of three shots: one at the first visit, one a month later, and the last six months after the second. Therefore, it takes at least six months before the body is protected from HAV and HBV, assuming all the doses have been given on schedule. Because it is possible to have more than one type of hepatitis, it is very important to vaccinate against infections that cause other types. However, there is no vaccine against hepatitis C.

Although most people who receive the HAV and HBV vaccines do develop effective immunity to these viruses, a small percent do not. You can ask to have your "HBV surface antibody" checked after you have received all doses of the vaccine. If the test shows that you do not have immunity, additional vaccine doses may stimulate you to make the needed antibodies. Unfortunately, a very small percent of people will never be able to mount an antibody response to the HBV vaccine.

If you lack immunity to either HAV or HBV and are exposed to either virus, there is another backup route to protection. Called immune globulin, it is administered through the vein. Immune globulin consists of the actual antibodies against the specific virus. If given early enough after exposure, immune globulin offers effective protection. HAV immune globulin can be given for up to 4 weeks after exposure but is probably effective only if given within 7 to 14 days after exposure. HBV immune globulin should also be given as soon as possible after the exposure and then repeated one month later. Again, there is no vaccine or specific immune globulin for HCV. Here are some recommendations for people with hepatitis:

- Drink absolutely no alcohol.
- Avoid high doses of Tylenol, aspirin, and non-steroidal anti-inflammatory medications such as Motrin, Advil, and Aleve (or prescription NSAIDs).
- Ask your primary care provider to vaccinate you against hepatitis A and B if blood tests show that you do not have the antibodies to these infections.
- If you do not have antibodies against hepatitis A, hepatitis B, or hepatitis C, avoid behaviors that can put you at risk for catching

these viruses, such as having unprotected sex or using injection drugs.

How Hepatitis Is Transmitted

Hepatitis A is transmitted through contaminated foods. Raw oysters in particular tend to carry infections like hepatitis A. But HBV and HCV travel quite differently. These viruses are transmitted the same way HIV is—through blood or sexual exposure. If you follow safe practices to avoid transmitting or catching HIV, you should theoretically be protecting yourself against catching HBV or HCV as well. However, unlike HIV, in some circumstances HBV can be very infectious, and a household contact may be at risk from a person who has a new HBV infection even if there is no blood or sexual contact. For this reason, your primary care provider may recommend that everyone in the house receive the HBV vaccine in certain situations. Blood used for transfusions is screened for HBV and HCV, so it is very rare to catch these infections today through a blood transfusion.

Hepatitis B Infection

Chronic HBV infection is a significant global disease affecting more than 350 million people worldwide. Fortunately, most adults infected with HBV are able to clear the infection within six months. Many people have no symptoms at all and only learn they were infected when their blood tests reveal a prior exposure. Fifteen to 40 percent of infected people develop complications including liver failure, cirrhosis, and liver cancer.

Blood Tests for HBV Infection

Blood is a complicated substance. It not only carries oxygen from the lungs to the tissues, but it also carries platelets to clot wounds, and immune system components like white blood cells and antibodies to fight infection. Laboratory blood tests can identify viral, bacterial, and fungal infections as well as disorders like anemia. The hepatitis blood tests check for viral "antigens" and hepatitis-specific "antibodies." *Antigens* are the proteins of the virus, and *antibodies* are the body's immune response to those proteins. Therefore, if your blood has never been exposed to the hepatitis B antigens, for example, it will not have any antibodies against hepatitis B, and your blood test will be negative for both HBV antigen and HBV antibodies. If you receive a vaccine against HBV and mount a full antibody response, your blood test will be negative for the antigen but positive for the antibody, and this will show that you are immune to HBV.

It should be noted that there are two types of antibodies commonly tested with regard to hepatitis B: the "core" antibody and the "surface" antibody. A positive *core* antibody results when a person has actually been infected by the hepatitis B virus, but a positive *surface* antibody may result either from the actual viral infection or when a person has only received the hepatitis B vaccine. The sequence and timeline for what happens with HBV infection is outlined in table 5.1.

Some people, especially those with weakened immune systems, are unable to clear their HBV infection; they become "chronic carriers."

Table 5.1
Timeline of Hepatitis B Infection

2–12 weeks	Blood tests show a positive HBV surface antigen and may also show a positive HBV e antigen.
5–15 weeks	The body has begun to make antibodies to the virus. Blood tests show a positive HBV core antibody (this generally turns positive before symptoms develop).
6–16 weeks	Symptoms may develop (this generally happens 4 weeks after the HBV surface antigen turns positive).
20+ weeks	The body works to make more antibodies. Blood tests show a positive HBV surface antibody if the immune system has mounted a good response to HBV.

Blood tests in these people will show a positive HBV surface antigen that persists after six months. The HBV "e" antigen is a second antigen often detected in people with a new HBV infection and is a very useful laboratory test because it can identify when a person's hepatitis is highly contagious. If blood tests persistently show a positive HBV e antigen, this means that the HBV is actively replicating and very contagious. Another way to determine whether the HBV is actively replicating is to test for the HBV genetic material or DNA.

Here is another blood test scenario: if you were infected with HBV and cleared your infection prior to having your blood test, your results would show a positive HBV core or surface antibody and a negative HBV surface antigen. This result would suggest that you are probably not contagious to others and that you probably do not have replicating HBV. However, this is only *probably*. A small percentage of people who have negative HBV surface antigens but positive core or surface antibodies *do* appear to have replicating HBV virus and may be infectious. So this test result would be somewhat reassuring, but not 100 percent. A summary of common HBV blood test results and their meanings is shown below in table 5.2.

Table 5.2
Interpreting HBV Blood Test Results

Blood test results	Clinical status	Infectious?
HBV surface antibody+ plus HBV surface antigen−	immunity from either vaccine or HBV infection	Not if immunity from vaccine; probably not if from HBV infection
HBV core antibody+ plus HBV surface antigen−	immunity from HBV infection	probably not
HBV surface antibody− plus HBV core antibody+ or HBV surface antibody− plus HBV surface antigen+	either acute infection or chronic carrier state	yes

Note: + means positive test results; − means negative test results.

HBV Treatments

The goal of hepatitis B treatment is to keep the virus from replicating. Effective medicines include Epivir (lamivudine), Roferon-A (interferon-alpha), and Intron-A (interferon-alpha). Eighty percent of people who respond to interferon-alpha lose their HBV surface antigen after completing therapy, and relapse is rare. Unfortunately, complications and side effects from this drug limit its use. Also, interferon-alpha must be given with a needle three times a week. A newer agent called Pegylated interferon-alpha (Peg-Intron or Pegasys) shows promise, however. It is a longer acting interferon and only needs to be given once per week. Pegylated interferon may be a more effective treatment for HBV than non-pegylated interferon because it maintains consistent and prolonged levels of interferon in the body rather than cycling through peaks and troughs the way non-pegylated interferon does. However, studies of pegylated interferon-alpha for HBV treatment have not been completed at this time.

Epivir is much easier to take than interferon-alpha and has few side effects. People with more severe liver inflammation appear to show the best response to Epivir. For this reason, Epivir treatment is mainly recommended for HBV chronic carriers who have replicating virus. The majority of people who take Epivir do achieve a response, but relapse is common when therapy is discontinued. Yet over time HBV can become resistant to Epivir treatment. This presents a dilemma. Experts don't know if it is better for people to stop taking their Epivir or to keep taking it if resistant strains of either HIV or HBV emerge. If the Epivir is discontinued, then the HBV infection may become more active. Emtriva or FTC is a HIV treatment that recently became available. Exacerbations of HBV infections have also been noted when patients stop Emtriva. The combination of interferon-alpha and Epivir has also been studied and appears to produce a higher rate of response than either medication used alone. The treatment of HBV with Emtriva has not been studied.

Two other promising medications used for HBV are Viread (tenofovir) and Hepsera (adefovir). Hepsera was first studied as a treatment for HIV, but it had so many side effects that it was not approved for this indication. However, very small doses of Hepsera do appear to be safe. These medications can be effective against HBV strains that have become resistant to Epivir.

Hepatitis C Infection

About 4 million Americans are estimated to have hepatitis C infection; probably about one third of HIV-infected individuals have HCV. The majority of people infected with HCV do not develop any symptoms at the time they become infected. About 15 percent resolve their infection within two years. The remaining 85 percent develop chronic infection. Twenty percent of people with chronic infection will progress to cirrhosis over a period of ten to twenty years. Unfortunately, people with HIV are more likely to progress to cirrhosis from their HCV disease than people without HIV. Other predictors for this outcome are a CD4 count less than 200, heavy alcohol consumption, and an age of less than 25 years at the time of HCV infection.

HCV Treatments

Not everyone infected with hepatitis C benefits from treatment. In some cases the side effects of treatment outweigh the possible benefits. Situations that would lead a primary care provider to advise *against* treatment are:

- Severe depression and not responding to treatment
- Severe anemia (low blood count) and not responding to treatment
- CD4 cell count below 200, since HCV treatment response will be poor
- Chest pain from heart disease while on medication
- Currently drinking alcohol or using drugs (people in methadone maintenance programs should still be eligible for HCV treatment)
- Pregnant or breast feeding

Many people with HCV, however, do benefit from treatment.

Once a person has been diagnosed with HCV infection, additional tests will be necessary to help shape treatment plans. These include routine liver function tests (which will show if the liver is inflamed), an HCV viral load test (which will determine if the HCV is active), an HCV genotype (which determines the "strain" of HCV), and a liver biopsy (to stage the extent of scarring or cirrhosis). Table 5.3 summarizes these tests, and table 5.4 lists those characteristics associated with the best response to treatment.

For hepatitis C, the preferred treatment is pegylated interferon-alpha (Peg-Intron or Pegasys) plus Rebetol (ribavirin)—usually for 48 weeks. Pegylated interferon-alpha is known to be more effective against HCV than non-pegylated interferon. Response to treatment is monitored by regular measuring of the HCV viral load and by repeated liver function tests. Sometimes a repeat liver biopsy may be helpful to demonstrate improvement in liver inflammation and scarring.

The best outcome for people who receive HCV treatment is called a "sustained response." This means that the HCV viral load is not detectable six months after treatment has been stopped. More than 95 percent of sustained responders continue to have nondetectable HCV viral load levels after years of follow-up. With the treatment regimen described above, the rate of sustained response may be as high as 30 to 50 percent for viral genotype 1, and 70 to 80 percent for non-1 genotypes of HCV. (Certain genotypes or strains of HCV respond better to treatment than others.) If relapse does occur and HCV viral load becomes detectable after treatment, a second round of treatment may yield a good response. However, chances for sustained response diminish if HCV treatment has already been tried once before.

Table 5.3

Considerations before Starting HCV Treatment

1. HCV viral load levels. If levels are very low, then treatment is not recommended.
2. HCV genotype or specific HCV strain can help predict responses to different treatments, if viral load levels are high enough to warrant any treatment.
3. Possibly a liver biopsy to see how much liver scarring is present.

Table 5.4

Predictors of a Good Response to HCV Treatment

1. Genotype 2 or 3
2. HCV viral load less than 2 million
3. No cirrhosis
4. Age 40 years or less
5. CD4 count over 200

Some people cannot take Rebetol (ribavirin) because of its side effects, and pregnant women should never take Rebetol. In addition, there is a theoretical question of whether there is a negative interaction between Rebetol and certain HIV treatments (Retrovir, Hivid, and Zerit), making the HIV treatments less effective. Therefore, these combinations should be used with caution. There is one combination, however, that we know should *not* be taken: Videx and Rebetol. If both of these medications are taken together, there is heightened risk for the rare side effect of "lactic acidosis," an increase in blood acid level, discussed in chapter 6. (People who cannot take Rebetol may get a response if they take only interferon-alpha, but rates of sustained response are low with non-pegylated interferon-alpha by itself, and Rebetol alone is ineffective for treatment.) Table 5.5 describes the side effects of HCV treatments.

Starting any treatment regimen for hepatitis C will change the quality of your life. It may be helpful to know what to expect. Most people who start treatment report fever, body aches, and flu-like symptoms. Headaches and fatigue are common. Also, treatment requires that you give yourself shots. Fortunately, the shots are very small and only need to be given once per week if you take the pegylated interferon. If your white blood cell count drops or if you become more anemic, however, your primary care provider may recommend specific medications that are also given as shots to boost the blood counts.

Milk thistle is an herbal remedy that has been promoted to protect the liver, but studies have not been done to find out whether it actually has any benefit. It may act by preventing the entry of liver toxins into healthy liver cells and by stimulating the production of new healthy

Table 5.5
Side Effects from HCV Treatments

Interferon-alpha
1. Fever and body aches (70% of people)
2. Depression (may worsen if you are already depressed)
3. Lower white blood cell and platelet* counts
4. Thyroid problems
5. Thinning hair

Ribavirin (Rebetol)
1. Anemia (low red blood cell count)
2. Gout
3. Severe effects on unborn babies if taken by pregnant women
4. Lactic acidosis (high blood acid level) if taken with Videx

* Platelets help the blood clot; low platelets can lead to easy bruising and bleeding.

cells. Toxic side effects from this herb have not been reported. However, milk thistle has been shown to slow the activity of a liver enzyme that metabolizes certain HIV treatments and methadone, thus raising the amounts of these drugs in the body above what has been prescribed. If you are on these treatments, you should avoid taking milk thistle until you have discussed it with your primary care provider, since dose adjustments may be necessary.

HIV and HCV treatments can be given at the same time, but the start of the therapies should be separated by two to three months. Unless liver disease is very severe, HIV treatments are generally started first. Ideally your immune system will improve with HIV treatments, your CD4 cell count will rise, and your body will be better equipped to mount a good response to HCV treatments.

Are there any options if your liver is severely damaged and doesn't respond to treatment? Liver transplants have been done in persons with HIV. A small study of twenty-three HIV-infected liver transplant recipients with a CD4 cell count over 200 who were on HIV treatments found their outcomes were similar to that in non-HIV-infected patients.

KEY POINTS

1. Some people have no symptoms at all from hepatitis, while others have nausea, vomiting, and stomach pain.

2. Hepatitis A, B, and C are diagnosed by blood tests. These tests also show whether the infection is new or chronic, and whether it is likely to be contagious.

3. If you have hepatitis, it is important to avoid both alcohol and common pain medications such as Tylenol, aspirin, and non-steroidal anti-inflammatory drugs like Motrin, Advil, and Aleve.

4. If you have hepatitis C and your blood tests show that you lack immunity to hepatitis A and B, you should receive hepatitis A and B vaccines.

5. Hepatitis A is usually acquired by eating contaminated food, but hepatitis B and C are transmitted through blood or sexual exposure.

6. Long-term complications from hepatitis B or C infections include liver failure, cirrhosis (irreversible scarring of the liver), and liver cancer.

7. Effective treatments for hepatitis B include interferon-alpha, Epivir (lamivudine), Viread (tenofovir), and Hepsera (adefovir).

8. The preferred treatment for hepatitis C is a combination of pegylated interferon-alpha and Rebetol (ribaviron). This treatment regimen can be very effective, especially for people treated for the first time.

Resources

1. HIV and Hepatitis.com at www.hivandhepatitis.com (information on hepatitis A, B, and C)

2. Center for Disease Control, Viral Hepatitis at www.cdc.gov/ncidod/diseases/hepatitis/ (information on hepatitis)

3. Medscape Resource Center: Hepatitis C at www.medscape.com/pages/editorial/resourcescenters/public/hepc/re-hepc.ov (information on hepatitis C with an emphasis on management)

4. National Library of Medicine Current Bibliographies in Medicine at www.nim.hih.gov/pubs/cbm/hepatitis_c_2002.html

6

Treatments for HIV

What treatments can control HIV?

When should HIV treatments be started?

When should HIV treatments be changed?

Can HIV treatments ever be stopped?

What HIV treatments are recommended for pregnant women?

When the HIV epidemic first emerged, the disease was poorly under-stood and seemed universally devastating. No targeted therapies were available, and health care providers did not have the tools they needed to monitor and fight the disease. But times have changed. This chapter describes the impressive arsenal of medications now employed to overpower HIV and preserve health. There is still no cure for HIV, but there are effective treatments.

Without question, these treatments are strong, but their strength against HIV carries the price tag of possible side effects and inconvenience. People who start HIV treatments must get used to taking pills on careful schedules and have to adjust to the routine of regular blood tests. In addition, the HIV treatments can not only bring side effects of their own, but they can also interact with other medications, making dose adjustments necessary. The decision of whether or when to start HIV treatments must be made with care. This chapter describes the available treatments and their side effects, along with guidelines for who should start therapy and when.

Antiretrovirals and Highly Active Antiretroviral Therapies: What Are They?

The potent medications that treat HIV infection are called "antiretroviral therapies." They work because they stop HIV from reproducing in the body. You can see the effect of these drugs by following your viral load level and CD4 cell count with blood tests (described in chapter 3). The aim of these medications is to decrease viral load levels while increasing CD4 cell counts.

Research on HIV continues, and new medications are being developed. Right now there are four dominant classes of HIV treatments on the market, each named for what it does to the virus: nucleoside or nucleotide reverse transcriptase inhibitors (RTIs); non-nucleoside reverse transcriptase inhibitors (NNRTIs); protease inhibitors (PIs); and fusion inhibitors (one category of entry inhibitors). Other entry inhibitors and integrase inhibitors are under study but not yet available. Each of these drugs interferes with HIV's ability to reproduce. The nucleoside, nucleotide, and non-nucleoside RTI drugs differ chemically but work on the same HIV enzyme (the reverse transcriptase). The other classes of drugs, PIs and fusion inhibitors, work on other targets in the life cycle of HIV to stop the virus from multiplying (see chapter 3 for a description of the HIV life cycle).

Years ago, providers treated HIV infection with just one or two HIV treatments, but it is now clear that the best results require at least three medications to be prescribed at once, including one or more very strong drugs. In general, the potent antiretrovirals include all of the PIs, all of the NNRTIs and one of the RTIs (only Ziagen or abacavir). A regimen containing three or more medications, including at least one potent therapy is called *highly active antiretroviral therapy*, or HAART. The term *combination therapy* has also been used.

When HAART is first given, most people enjoy seeing their viral load drop to levels that cannot be detected by blood tests (that is, below 50). Although you can see amazing results in less than three weeks, it can sometimes take from three to six months to drive the viral load down to the lowest level. Be aware that HAART regimens are expensive. The monthly costs of RTIs, NNRTIs, and PIs are approximately $200, $250, and $500, respectively. The cost of Fuzeon, the one currently available fusion inhibitor, is $20,000 a year. Fortunately, assistance programs usually cover the costs of these treatments for people without insurance.

Important Things to Know When Starting Treatment

A virus, like a person, is resourceful. When blocked in one direction, it will try to go around in another. When a drug stops a necessary enzyme, for example, a virus will try to reproduce without that enzyme. It will change. These changes, called "mutations," explain why drugs sometimes lose their power. New strains of virus can emerge, challenging scientists to develop drugs with different target enzymes or with different mechanisms of action. This problem affects antibiotics and antiretrovirals. We are always trying to stay a few steps ahead of the virus.

If you have never taken HIV treatments before, you are less likely to be infected with a virus that has mutations. However, when people have taken several HIV treatments, they are at greater risk for becoming infected with a drug-resistant virus—one that has undergone many mutations. This makes sense, because any nonresistant virus would have been stopped by the drugs, leaving only the resistant strains to reproduce. The goal is to keep your viral load very low on treatment so that there are few copies of the virus in your system and therefore few working to develop resistance. This is a very desirable situation.

On the other hand, a high viral load in the bloodstream means that there are viruses working to develop resistance, and the risk of effective mutations is higher. In this situation, there is a reasonable likelihood that the HIV will become resistant to one or all of the treatments it is facing. For this reason, it is critical to take all the doses of all the treatments. If, for example, a person took only one of the prescribed treatments or took only some of the doses or pills, the drug effect is much weaker. The viral load will increase, with many viruses working to develop mutations, and the odds of a drug-resistant strain emerging are greatly increased. *This can happen if you miss as little as one to two doses a week.*

When considering whether to start or change HIV treatments, take into account the following important points:

1. Your best chance for getting your viral load down to very low levels happens when you first start taking treatments because the virus is most likely still sensitive to all the medicines. It is a terrible shame when people waste this window of opportunity by starting HIV treatments without being seriously committed to following their treatment regimens exactly as prescribed. This cannot be emphasized strongly enough. *It is extremely important that you be mentally ready to start treatment before you actually start, because without good follow-through, the virus is likely to become drug-resistant.*

2. You should take the HIV treatments as prescribed and make sure you understand all of the directions you have received. If you are unsure about the dosing, you should talk to your primary care provider immediately. No question is a stupid question. These regimens are complicated, and it is always smart to ask as many questions as it takes until you feel confident about what your treatment plan requires. Your provider *expects* you to repeat questions, and your provider *expects* to go over the same information with you more than once.

3. If you cannot immediately reach your primary care provider in an emergency (for example, if you are vomiting), it is better to take *none* of the HIV treatments than to take partial doses. Even if the viral load goes up, HIV cannot become resistant to the treatments if you are not taking them.

4. It is important to be honest with your primary care provider. If your viral load goes up, your provider needs to know if this is because

the HIV has become resistant or if it is because you are having trouble taking the medicines as prescribed. There is absolutely nothing to be gained by deceiving your primary care provider, and there is no shame in having difficulty managing HIV treatment.

5. There are several HIV treatments available and many things to consider when developing a treatment regimen. How strong are the pills? What are their side effects? How often do the pills need to be taken? And how many pills need to be taken at one time? The daily number of pills required can range from one pill twice a day to more than twenty pills per day, divided into either two or three doses. Your primary care provider may advise against certain medications because of their side effects or because they may be less effective against certain HIV strains. You should discuss all options with your provider and together determine which medication regimen will work best for you.

National Guidelines for Starting and Changing HIV Treatments in Nonpregnant People

HIV experts from three groups have developed treatment guidelines used by health care providers throughout the world. These groups are the Department of Health and Human Services (DHHS), the International AIDS Society–USA Panel (IAS-USA), and the British HIV Association. DHHS guidelines are available on the Web at www .aidsinfo.nih.gov/guidelines or www.cdcnpin.org. The HIV experts who prepared these guidelines relied on data from studies that have compared outcomes for people taking different HIV treatments over the years. This information has helped clarify when it makes the most sense to start or change treatments. Recommendations are slightly different for pregnant women and are discussed in chapter 11. The recommendations from the three groups for nonpregnant adults and adolescents are similar and, for certain populations, are in absolute agreement. Table 6.1 summarizes the three groups' shared recommendations on when to start HIV treatments and when to wait.

Sometimes the advantages of treatment clearly outweigh the advantages of waiting, and sometimes it clearly seems better to wait. For

Table 6.1
HIV Treatment Recommendations for Nonpregnant Adults and Adolescents

---

HIV treatment is definitely recommended when:
- a person is symptomatic*
- a person's CD4 cell count is below 200

HIV treatment may be recommended when:
- a person is symptom-free, with a CD4 cell count between 200 and 350 and a low viral load level**
- a person is symptom-free, with a CD4 cell count greater than 350, but with a high viral load level**

HIV treatment can probably be safely postponed when:
- a person is symptom-free, with a CD4 cell count greater than 350 and a low viral load level**

---

* HIV-related symptoms are discussed in chapter 4.
** Department of Health and Human Services (DHHS) guidelines advise the consideration of HIV treatments when viral load levels reach 55,000 or above.

some people, however, the decision is less clear-cut: people who have both a high viral load and a high CD4 count, or who have both a low viral load and a low CD4 count of 200 to 350. This "middle group" may do well either to start treatment or to wait; studies have not strongly indicated a recommendation in either direction. However, all experts agree that the most important qualification to starting treatment is that you be mentally prepared for the commitment, regardless of your numbers. If you fit into the middle category, it is important to discuss the pros and cons of starting HIV treatments with your provider and to take time to make your decision.

The DHHS guidelines published in July 2003 advise nonpregnant, asymptomatic people with HIV to consider treatment when CD4 counts drop below 350 and/or viral loads exceed either 55,000 (by the PCR method or bDNA method). People who are experiencing HIV-related symptoms, however, are advised to start on HIV treatments regardless of CD4 cell count and viral load levels. The guidelines are updated periodically; you may wish to consult the Web sites (aidsinfo.nih.gov/guidelines or www.cdcnpin.org) to access the most recent version.

Recent studies have brought to light another factor that can affect treatment plans for women: when measured at the same CD4 count, viral loads seem to be lower in women with HIV than in men with HIV if the CD4 count is over 200. In other words, if a woman and a man both have the same CD4 count, it is probable that the woman's viral load will be lower than the man's. This observation does not imply that women get sick at a different rate than men do, but it does suggest that women may benefit from starting HIV treatment at lower viral load levels than those specified in the guidelines.

Should You Begin HIV Treatment?

The ultimate decision of when to start treatment is up to you, regardless of the numbers. It is a difficult decision that thousands of people have struggled with. Talking with other people who have wrestled with this choice can be enormously helpful. Your health care provider should be able to connect you with support groups. There is no simple answer. Important considerations to weigh as you make this decision are outlined in table 6.2.

HIV Treatment Names

If you decide that you are ready to start treatment, your primary care provider should explain the value of combining at least three HIV treatments—a HAART regimen—sometimes referred to as a "cocktail." As discussed in the previous section, the combination should include at least one very strong or potent medication. The only people advised to take just one antiretroviral medication (monotherapy) rather than a combination of drugs are pregnant women with high CD4 cell counts and very low viral loads. For this population, Retrovir alone is an option. Note that chapter 11 focuses on HIV and pregnancy. The guidelines discussed below apply to people who are not pregnant.

Table 6.2
Benefits and Risks of Waiting to Start HIV Treatment

Benefits of waiting:
- You can postpone the inconvenience and chore of taking medications
- You can postpone medication-related side effects
- No drug resistance can develop when you are not taking medicines
- You preserve more future choices for antiretroviral medications if you should later get sick from HIV

Risks of waiting:
- You may face immune system damage that won't ever improve
- You may have more difficulty in decreasing the viral load level
- You may have a higher risk of transmitting HIV to others

Adapted from table 4 in "Guidelines for the Use of Antiretroviral Agents in HIV-Infected Adults and Adolescents—November 10, 2003" http://aidsinfo.nih.gov/guidelines/.

The particular regimens proposed in the guidelines were developed with consideration of combined drug strength, daily number of pills, side effects, and convenience. Before looking at the specific regimens, be aware that medication names are often confusing because almost all drugs have two names: first, the generic or scientific name, and second, the brand name. Some medications are also referred to by abbreviations. The ins and outs of this system may become clearer by referring to table 6.3, which pairs the two different names for each medication.

Recommended HIV Treatment Regimens
Persons Who Are Starting Treatment for the First Time, or "ARV-Naive" Patients

For many people, the decision to start HIV treatment involves a transition from life without any regular pills to life with what seems like a shocking number of pills. Pharmacies sell simple plastic boxes that have separate compartments for each day of the week so that pills can be sorted in advance. Your primary care provider may also be able to

Table 6.3
HIV Treatment Names and Classes

Generic name	Abbreviation	Trade name	What does it look like?*
Nucleoside or Nucleotide Reverse Transcriptase Inhibitors (RTIs)			
Zidovudine	AZT, ZDV	Retrovir	white round tablet
Didanosine	ddI	Videx	large white round tablet
Zalcitibine	ddC	Hivid	small blue capsule
Stavudine	d4T	Zerit	brown capsule
Lamivudine	3TC	Epivir	small white diamond tablet
Lamivudine/ Zidovudine	AZT/3TC	Combivir	white oblong tablet
Abacavir		Ziagen	oblong yellow tablet
Lamivudine/ Zidovudine/ Abacavir		Trizivir	blue oblong tablet
Emtricitabine	FTC	Emtriva	blue and white capsule
Viread		Tenofovir	light blue oblong tablet
Non-Nucleoside Reverse Transcriptase Inhibitors (NNRTIs)			
Nevirapine		Virammune	white oblong tablet
Delavirdine		Rescriptor	white oblong tablet
Efavirenz		Sustiva	brown capsule
Protease Inhibitors (PIs)			
Saquinavir		Fortivase	large tan capsule
Ritonavir		Norvir	large white capsule
Indinavir		Crixivan	white capsule
Nelfinavir		Viracept	oblong blue tablet
Amprenavir		Agenerase	large white capsule
Lopinavir/Ritonavir		Kaletra	large orange capsule
Atazanavir		Reyataz	blue capsule
Fosamprenavir		Lexiva	white oblong tablet
Fusion Inhibitor			
Enfuvirtide	T-20	Fuzeon	injectable

* If the pills you receive when you refill a prescription look different from how the pill is described here or from the last time you filled the prescription, check with your provider and make sure you received the proper medication.

provide you with a pill organizer. Organizing pills and pill schedules is very important because missed doses can increase the chance of drug resistance.

Health care providers know how difficult it is to keep track of so many pills, especially when some need to be taken with food, some without, some once a day, and some many times a day. It is very important to plan how and when each medicine will be taken and to understand the requirements of each. It is also important to know yourself. For example, some people want to take their pills in private, and this can be challenging at school or work. Sometimes it is helpful to do a "trial run" of the planned regimen by substituting different colored M&Ms or jelly beans for the different medicines. Watch alarms or alarm clocks are often used as reminders of when to take daily doses. Household members or reliable friends may also be available to help with reminders and to give daily encouragement. If you stick to your regimen, the rewarding increase in your CD4 cell count and the decrease in your viral load will also serve to reinforce the value of your commitment.

Now let's consider the actual regimens. The DHHS guidelines published in July 2003 recommend "preferred" and "alternative" regimens for three "class-based" regimens: NNRTI-based regimens, PI-based regimens, and triple NRTI regimens in initiating therapy for persons who have never previously been treated with HIV treatments (or "ARV-naive persons"). The NNRTI-based regimens have been compared to PI-based regimens, and all regimens are very effective in decreasing viral load levels and maintaining low values.

The first study of the triple NRTI regimen found it equally effective as a PI-based regimen (Crixivan was the PI used in the study), but persons with baseline high viral loads over 100,000 on the triple NRTI regimen were less likely to maintain a low viral load when compared to persons on the PI-based regimen. A recent study found persons on the triple NRTI regimen were more likely to have rises in their viral loads over time (meaning the HIV treatments were no longer working for them) when compared to persons on a Sustiva-based regimen. Even though the triple NRTI regimen may not be quite as strong as the NNRTI- or PI-based regimens, there are still advantages to triple

NRTI regimens, including the simplicity and low number of pills, fewer interactions with other drugs, and perhaps less worrisome side effects. *For these reasons, the DHHS guidelines recommend that the triple NRTI regimen be used as an alternative to the NNRTI- or PI-based regimens only for persons with baseline viral loads of less than 100,000.*

The actual recommendations outlined in table 6.4 can also be found at www.aidsinfo.nih.gov/guidelines/. The recommendations were written prior to the availability of Reyataz, Lexiva, and Emtriva, so these medications are not included in the guidelines. *Sustiva is not recommended for pregnant women or women who may become pregnant because of side effects to the fetus.* Additional information on HIV treatments in pregnancy is discussed in chapter 11.

With the exception of offering Retrovir as the only HIV treatment

Table 6.4
Class-Based Regimens Recommended by DHHS (July 2003)

Class-based regimen		Number of pills/ day
NNRTI-Based		
Preferred	Sustiva + Epivir + (Retrovir or Viread or Zerit)	3–5 pills
Alternatives	Sustiva + Epivir + Videx	3–5 pills
	Virammune + Epivir + (Retrovir or Viread or Zerit)	4–6 pills
PI-Based		
Preferred	Kaletra + Epivir + (Retrovir or Zerit)	8–10 pills
Alternatives	Agenerase + Norvir* + Epivir + (Retrovir or Zerit)	12–14 pills
	Crixivan +/− Norvir* + Epivir + (Retrovir or Zerit)	8–12 pills
	Viracept + Epivir + (Retrovir or Zerit)	6–14 pills
	Fortivase + Norvir* + Epivir + (Retrovir or Zerit)	14–16 pills
	Invirase + Norvir* + Epivir + (Retrovir or Zerit)	14–16 pills
Triple NRTI Regimens (alternative to NNRTI- or PI-based regimens)		
	Ziagen + Epivir + (Retrovir or Zerit)	2–6 pills

* Norvir is given only as a low dose, or 100 to 400 mg/day, to boost the levels of the second PI.

to pregnant women with very low viral loads and high CD4 cell counts, monotherapy (taking only one HIV treatment), should never be a choice. Even taking only two HIV treatments together is not recommended because it is clear they are not strong enough to keep the virus under control. Hydrea is not a HIV treatment, but it can make certain HIV treatments, such as Videx, stronger. However, Hydrea is no longer recommended to be included in treatment regimens because of possible severe side effects. Additional HIV treatments or combinations that should be avoided or never used in regimens for patients starting therapy for the first time, or "ARV-naive" patients, are:

- Rescriptor (weaker than recommended options)
- Retrovir + Hivid (weaker than recommended options)
- Invirase as only PI (weaker than recommended options)
- Agenerase as only PI (too many pills)
- Fortivase as only PI (too many pills)
- Viracept + (Fortivase or Invirase) (too many pills)
- Norvir as the only PI (more side effects than recommended options)
- Zerit + Videx (more and worse side effects than recommended options, use in pregnancy only if benefits outweigh risks)
- Hivid + Zerit (more side effects than recommended options)
- Hivid + Videx (more side effects than recommended options)
- Retrovir + Zerit (the interaction makes the drugs work against each other)
- Sustiva in pregnancy (side effects to fetus)
- Reyataz + Crixivan (possible worse side effects)
- Viread + Epivir + Ziagen or Videx (high treatment failure rate)
- Emtriva + Epivir (similar resistance profile)

There still are many options. How do you decide? Your primary care provider will probably list the choices he or she thinks are best for you, which may not include every regimen listed above. Some aspects to consider in comparing the regimens include number of pills, number of doses a day, food requirements, and which side effects you can live with. Today patients have both more options and better options than patients starting HIV treatments before 1995 had.

Once-Daily Therapy

Once-daily therapy is now an option. HIV treatments that are approved for once-daily therapy by the Food and Drug Administration (FDA) include Sustiva, Videx, Viread, Epivir, Zerit extended release, Emtriva, Reyataz, and the combination of Agenerase or Lexiva + low dose Norvir. Although not yet approved, once-daily dosing of other PIs boosted with low doses of Norvir (including Kaletra) and Virammune have also been studied. However, the only drug with a very long half life is Sustiva, which means it is less concerning if you delay or miss a dose because you will still have some Sustiva in your blood. Missing doses of the other drugs means probably having very low or absent doses in your blood, which can lead to the virus becoming resistant.

Dosing and Food Requirements

It would be ideal if HIV treatment were as simple as taking one daily vitamin tablet. Unfortunately, the most effective treatment, combination therapy, gets rather complicated. On the bright side, it usually does not involve daily injections or trips to the clinic. All it demands is careful planning, good pill management, and genuine commitment.

Table 6.5 outlines the food requirements and dosing for each medication. Why does food matter? The presence or absence of food in your stomach can influence the amount of medication absorbed from a given dose. Some medicines are best absorbed with food, and some are more effective when taken on an empty stomach. (Fortunately, there are also many drugs that have no special food requirements at all.) These food recommendations are important, *but not more important than the dosing schedule.* Therefore, if a particular medicine is supposed to be taken with food and you have no food at the right time, you should still take the medicine. It is better to have low levels, as opposed to no levels, of med-

Table 6.5
Antiretroviral Food Requiremen

Medication	Food requirement	
Retrovir	No food requirement	
Videx	Empty stomach	
Hivid	No food requirement	
Zerit	No food requirement	
Epivir	No food requirement	
Ziagen	No food requirement, but alcohol increases levels 41%	1 pill twice daily
Emtriva	No food requirement	1 pill once daily
Viread	Take with food	1 pill once daily
Virammune	No food requirement	1 pill twice daily
Rescriptor	No food requirement	6 pills twice daily
Sustiva	No food requirement	3 pills daily
Crixivan	Empty stomach or skim milk or low fat meal	2 pills three times daily
Norvir	Take with food	6 pills twice daily
Viracept	Take with food	5 pills twice daily
Fortivase	Take with food	8 pills twice daily
Agenerase	Avoid high-fat meals, but otherwise can take with or without food	8 pills twice daily
Kaletra	Take with food	3 pills twice daily
Reyataz	Take with food	2 pills once daily
Lexiva	No food requirement	2 pills twice daily
Fuzeon	No food requirement	injected twice daily

Partial text visible in torn corner: ication. Likewis / empty-stom / While / pers / ki

* Most frequently used dosing. Some medications are given less often to people with kidney problems. Some medications may also be given at lower doses and less frequently if prescribed together (for example, using Norvir with many of the PIs will decrease the number of doses and pills).

, if you accidentally ate just before the time to take an
ch medicine, you should still take it.

common doses of each drug are listed in table 6.5, your own
al dosing will depend on your weight and on the health of your
dneys. Though most of the studies behind typical dosing guidelines
were based on trials of men, not women, it is not thought that women
require significantly different guidelines. However, blood levels of one
drug, Rescriptor, do appear to be higher in women—but there are no
special dosing guidelines for women.

Lab Tests after Starting HIV Treatment

The ideal goal of antiretroviral therapy is to overwhelm the virus, to
stop it from reproducing, and to make it undetectable in the blood by
reducing the viral load to less than 50. This does happen. Between two
and six weeks after starting therapy, your primary care provider will
draw a viral load level, hoping for a result below 400. A substantial,
even threefold drop in the original level should not be surprising. The
goal load of less than 400 (or even less than 50) is generally met within
three months of starting therapy, but it can take up to a year. Fifty to
90 percent of people who have never been on HIV treatments before
are able to achieve these low viral loads.

Once the viral load level drops to less than 50, your provider will
likely check it every three months. If it rises, you will probably be asked
to repeat the test to be sure that the rise is a true rise. Sometimes the
viral load can "blip" up and then fall again. But if the viral load is truly
rising, and you have been taking your HIV treatments faithfully, it may
mean that the HIV has become resistant to the particular medications
you are taking.

In addition to the viral load tests, there are separate blood tests to
monitor for viral resistance to treatments. It takes a couple of weeks to
get results from the most common of these tests, called a *genotype test*.
This test looks for changes (called *mutations*) that might be taking place
in the virus. The genotype test looks at the reverse transcriptase and
protease genes, or genetic material.

The second blood test is called a *phenotype test*. This test takes longer and can be more difficult to order. Phenotype testing reveals what concentration of each medicine is required to prevent the virus from multiplying. To do a phenotype test, the laboratory inserts the pattern or sequence of the reverse transcriptase and protease gene from the patient's HIV strain into an HIV strain that the laboratory uses. The laboratory then measures how well this laboratory HIV strain can reproduce or multiply when antiretroviral treatments are added.

Both genotype and phenotype tests are expensive, and neither test is routinely ordered in people who have never before taken HIV treatments. In some areas of the country, however, people are more likely to be infected with viruses that are already resistant to certain drugs; and in those circumstances, the primary care provider finds it helpful to have genotype results before selecting the first HIV treatment regimen. Genotype testing is recommended when someone does not respond to or fails their first treatment regimen, as well as during acute HIV infection.

A third population, pregnant women, may also warrant genotype testing. Because the risk of transmitting HIV to an unborn baby is highest when viral loads are high (see chapter 11), it is especially important to decrease viral loads as rapidly as possible in pregnancy. The International AIDS Society–USA Panel and EuroGuidelines Group for HIV Resistance recently recommended that all pregnant women with detectable viral loads undergo resistance testing.

It is difficult to run any resistance testing if the viral load is less than 1,000.

Persons Who Are Changing Treatments, or "ARV-Experienced" Patients

If you are no longer responding to your HIV treatment, your primary care provider will likely do the following:

- Review every HIV treatment that you have ever taken
- Do a physical exam to check for new findings that may be related to the HIV becoming active

- Discuss how well you are taking the medications (for example, do you miss doses?)
- Review all other medications that you may be on to check for drug interactions that may lower the blood levels of your HIV treatments
- Perform resistance testing

If it is clear that you are taking every dose of every HIV treatment and there are no possible drug interactions, your primary care provider may add an additional HIV treatment, change one to two of the HIV treatments, or change the entire regimen to a new regimen. Different strategies depending on the scenario are described below.

Scenario 1. If you have been on your current regimen for a limited period of time and your viral load level has substantially decreased to less than 5,000 but over 50, your primary care provider may consider "intensification," that is, making your regimen stronger with an additional HIV treatment such as Viread, or making one of your HIV treatments stronger, such as boosting a PI in your regimen or increasing the PI blood levels by adding a small dose of Norvir. Intensification would not be a good strategy if you initially responded to your current regimen, then had your viral load rise several months or years later. This pattern suggests your virus has become resistant to one or more HIV treatments in your regimen and it would be better to change the HIV treatments.

Scenario 2. If resistance testing identifies that your virus is resistant to one or more of the HIV treatments that you are taking, your primary care provider may choose to change just the one or two drugs that will not work for you or may change the whole regimen. The new HIV treatments would be ones to which your virus should be susceptible, based on the resistance testing. If you have resistance to more than one treatment, your primary care provider will probably put you on a HIV treatment from another class (for example, if you were on a PI, you could change to a NNRTI, or vice versa).

Scenario 3. If your resistance testing shows no resistance, your primary care provider will probably go over your regimen again to be sure you are taking it correctly. They may consider starting a new regimen and doing resistance testing again in 2 to 4 weeks.

Scenario 4. If your virus is very resistant and you have no or just a few options, your primary care provider may keep you on your current regimen if you appear to be getting some benefit. If possible, you want to avoid adding a single active HIV treatment because your virus will probably develop resistance quickly. If your virus is only sensitive to one or two available HIV treatments, your primary care provider may want to wait until one or two additional new treatments become available either through FDA approval or through a study (see chapter 19 for discussion on research studies). Other strategies you and your primary care provider can consider include the following:

- Boosting or raising the levels of some PIs with low doses of Norvir
- Checking blood levels of specific HIV treatments to be sure they are adequate (*therapeutic drug monitoring*)
- Using several HIV treatments (including up to 3 PIs or 2 NNRTIs) in the hope that the virus has some sensitivity to some of the treatments
- Trying old HIV treatments again, particularly if you stopped them previously because of side effects

Fuzeon, or T-20, is the first drug in a new class of HIV treatments and appears very promising for persons who have limited treatment options. Given the need to give this treatment by a shot twice a day and the possibility of side effects related to receiving shots, Fuzeon is recommended only for persons who have already received several HIV treatments, or "ARV-experienced" patients.

HIV Treatment Side Effects

Fortunately, most people who start HIV treatment do not have serious side effects from their medicines. But even nonserious side effects can be unpleasant. In developing a treatment plan with your health care provider, the goal will be to find an effective regimen that also leaves you feeling well. To do this, you will have to weigh the possible side effects of different medications and choose those that are the least worrisome to you. No medication can guarantee a total absence of possible side effects—and that includes over-the-counter medicines as well as prescription drugs. Reading descriptions of potential side effects is never fun, but it is important to have this information before choosing your regimen. As you consider the following explanations of various side effects, remember that these are *possibilities*, not inevitable consequences.

Tables 6.6 and 6.7 summarize the most common side effects associated with HIV treatments. These include nausea, headache, rash, diarrhea, nerve pain, and inflammation of the liver or pancreas. Other possible side effects may be less familiar than those described in the tables. Three additional side effects that you should be aware of are:

Table 6.6
Most Common Side Effects of HIV Treatment Not Including "Metabolic" Side Effects

Antiretroviral	Common side effects
Retrovir	low blood cell counts (such as anemia*), nausea, headache, inflamed muscles
Videx	nausea, diarrhea, neuropathy,* pancreatitis*
Hivid	neuropathy,* pancreatitis,* mouth ulcers
Zerit	neuropathy,* pancreatitis,* headache, nausea
Epivir	headache, nausea
Combivir	see Retrovir/Epivir
Ziagen	allergic reaction,** nausea
Trizivir	see Retrovir/Epivir/abacavir
Emtriva	headache, diarrhea, nausea, rash
Viread	nausea, vomiting, diarrhea, intestinal gas
Virammune	rash (may be more common in women), hepatitis,* nausea
Rescriptor	rash, hepatitis,* nausea

Table 6.6 (*continued*)

Antiretroviral	Common side effects
Sustiva	dizziness, nightmares, headache, rash, trouble sleeping, depression, nausea, hepatitis
Fortivase	diarrhea, nausea, headache, tiredness
Norvir	nausea, tingling around the mouth, bad aftertaste, headache, diarrhea
Crixivan	kidney stones, nausea, yellowing of the skin or eyes***
Viracept	diarrhea, nausea
Agenerase	nausea, rash, other****
Kaletra	nausea, diarrhea, headache
Reyataz	yellowing of the skin or eyes,*** changes in the way the heart beats, worsening of liver disease (for example, if you have hepatitis B or C)
Lexiva	diarrhea, nausea, rash
Fuzeon	allergic reactions, injection site reactions, possibly higher risk for pneumonia

Note: The side effects listed here do not include the "metabolic" side effects such as fat maldistribution, increases in blood sugar, increases in blood fats, and increases in blood acid levels. These side effects have been associated with nearly all HIV treatments. (See further discussion in this chapter.)

* Neuropathy and anemia are discussed in chapter 4; hepatitis is discussed in chapter 5. Pancreatitis, inflammation of the pancreas, can be serious and require hospitalization; its symptoms include abdominal pain, nausea, and vomiting.

** Approximately 4% of patients may have an allergic reaction that has at least two symptoms. The most common symptoms are rash, fever, and muscle aches. Other symptoms include lung or gastrointestinal complaints. In allergic reactions, symptoms get worse with every dose of Ziagen (abacavir). Most reactions occur within 11 days. If you have an allergic reaction to Ziagen you should never take the drug again because it could be life-threatening.

*** The yellowing of the eyes and skin may be due to increases in bilirubin levels in the blood. Bilirubin results from the turnover of red blood cells through the liver. This side effect is not serious and does not necessarily mean you have liver disease if the high bilirubin is due to HIV treatments. The yellowing will not damage your skin or eyes and should go away after you stop the treatment.

**** The liquid solution of Agenerase contains propylene glycol, which should not be taken by pregnant women, children younger than four years old, people with liver or kidney problems, or anyone taking antiabuse Flagyl.

Table 6.7

Most Common HIV Treatment Side Effects and What May Cause Them

Common side effect	Possible cause
Nausea	All HIV treatments, but especially Videx, Viread, Fortivase, Norvir, Crixivan, Agenerase, Kaletra
Diarrhea	Videx, Viread, Fortivase, Viracept, Kaletra, Lexiva
Neuropathy	Videx, Hivid, Zerit
Pancreatitis	Videx, Hivid, Zerit
Hepatitis	Nearly all HIV treatments, especially Virammune, Rescriptor, Sustiva
Rash	Nearly all HIV treatments, especially Virammune, Rescriptor, Sustiva, Agenerase, Ziagen Lexiva
Headache	Nearly all HIV treatments, especially Retrovir, Epivir, Sustiva
Yellowing of skin or eyes	Crixivan, Reyataz
Fat maldistribution	Possibly all HIV treatments
Elevated blood sugar	Protease inhibitors
Elevated blood fat levels	Protease inhibitors, particularly Norvir, less likely with Reyataz
Elevated blood acid levels	Nucleoside or possibly nucleotide reverse transcriptase inhibitors, particularly the combination of Zerit and Videx

Note: Neuropathy is discussed in chapter 4. Hepatitis is discussed in chapter 5. Pancreatitis can be a serious condition requiring hospitalization; the symptoms of pancreatitis include abdominal pain, nausea, and vomiting.

(1) changes in body shape, also referred to as lipodystrophy or fat maldistribution; (2) increases in blood sugar, also known as diabetes; and (3) increases in blood fat, also called hyperlipidemia.

The terms *lipodystrophy* and *fat maldistribution* have been used to describe body shape changes that appear to be associated with HIV treatments. However, these redistributions of fat have also been seen in people who have never taken HIV treatments. People may feel as if their fat has shifted around. When this happens, fat is usually lost from the face and legs and gained in the belly, breasts, or elsewhere. One location for fat growth that some people find particularly troublesome is at the top of the back and behind the neck (commonly and unflatteringly called "a buffalo hump"). Women who have fat maldistribution are most likely to complain of a big stomach, larger breasts, and thinner legs. Women tend to gain more fat than they lose. Some women think they look pregnant. While these changes are cosmetically troubling, the one of most medical concern is the increase in waist size, since this finding in the HIV-negative population has been associated with a higher risk of heart disease, diabetes, stroke, gallstones, and breast cancer.

It's not clear what causes fat maldistribution. Changes in body shape seem to be more common in older people and in those who have taken HIV treatments for a long time. Yet because the benefits of HIV treatment far outweigh the problems associated with body fat changes, experts do not recommend that treatments be stopped in people who develop lipodystrophy. What can be done about the possible risks of this side effect? Protect yourself with healthy lifestyle choices. Do not smoke. Cigarettes are associated with a significantly increased risk of stroke, heart disease, and cancer. Eat a low fat and low sugar diet. Exercise to improve muscle tone and general health. Certain medicines like Serostatin (human growth hormone) and anabolic therapies such as Anadrol (oxymetholone) or Oxandrin (oxandrolone) may have some benefit, but they require further study. Sometimes minor surgery can also help, especially for fat pads on the neck if they are uncomfortable. Generally stopping or changing HIV treatments is not helpful, but some persons have noted an improvement in how they look.

The second important side effect to consider is diabetes, which refers to increased levels of sugar in the blood. (Standard blood work includes measuring sugar, called glucose monitoring.) Diabetes is very common in the United States, and most people who have diabetes are not infected with HIV. Starting PIs can worsen any tendencies you may have to develop diabetes. If your sugar levels run high prior to starting HIV treatment and you have the option, it may be wise for you to choose a regimen that does not include a PI. The first treatment for high blood sugar is a special diet. If this fails to control the sugar level, there are several medication choices, including both pills and insulin shots.

The third side effect, increased fat levels, sometimes requires medical treatment if adjustments to diet fail to reduce the levels. PIs are known to increase the blood levels of three kinds of fat: triglycerides, total cholesterol, and low-density lipoprotein or LDH (see chapter 13 for further discussion on fat levels). Your provider should routinely check these levels if you are on HIV treatments. Because these tests require you to avoid all food for approximately 12 hours before your blood is drawn, it is a good idea to check in advance if these (or any other) "fasting blood tests" are planned so that you can arrange to have your blood drawn first thing in the morning. For more about heart health, see chapter 13.

Studies that have looked at differences between men and women in the side effects of HIV treatment have found that women are more likely than men to have severe skin rashes and hepatitis due to Virammune and that women may be more likely in general to develop hepatitis due to any HIV treatment.

Finally, one recently noticed yet rare side effect is called "lactic acidosis." It seems to be related to nucleoside reverse transcriptase inhibitors, particularly the combination of Zerit and Videx. The first study describing this condition found that women were more likely to be affected by it than men. People with lactic acidosis may have nausea, vomiting, and stomach pain. Their blood work may show an inflamed liver and a high level of acid. Some women also develop lung or kidney problems. Pregnant women taking both Videx and Zerit and anyone taking both Rebetol and Videx appear to be at particular risk for lactic acidosis, and these combinations should be avoided.

Taking HIV Treatments with Other Medications

Because all medicines mix in the body, there is always the chance that they will interact with each other. Consider the examples of "Drug A" and "Drug B." If Drug A interferes with the breakdown of Drug B, a higher amount of Drug B will linger in the body than if Drug A had not also been taken. On the other hand, if Drug A *accelerates* the breakdown of Drug B, then too little Drug B will circulate in the body as a result. Some drug interactions can be dangerous to health. Sometimes, however, two drugs can work together "synergistically," which means that each drug helps the other work to its highest potential.

One common example of two drugs working synergistically together is Norvir and some other PIs. Using a small dose of Norvir "boosts" or raises the blood level of other selected PIs. In fact, Kaletra is a combination of lopinavir and Norvir. Some "boosted" PIs may have such good blood levels that they may need to be taken just once a day. Another example of drugs interacting together is the combination of Videx and Viread. A lower dose of Videx can probably be used if it is taken with Viread. However, Viread or Sustiva will lower the dose of Reyataz, so Norvir should be added to the regimen to boost the Reyataz levels.

Because drug interactions are complicated, researchers have paid a great deal of attention to them. Certain drug interactions are so common that they have become predictable. Problems can be avoided when the person writing your prescriptions has a clear list of every medicine that you take, including over-the-counter medicines. HIV treatments are known to interact with several other drugs. For example, methadone decreases levels of Videx and Sustiva. Virammune, Norvir, Viracept, and Kaletra all decrease levels of methadone.

Birth control pills also interact with HIV medications (especially with the NNRTIs and PIs). The only protease inhibitors that do *not* significantly interact with oral contraceptive pills are Crixivan and Reyataz (atazanavir). Taken with any other antiretroviral treatments, birth control pills become unreliable. If you are taking both oral contraceptives and either a protease inhibitor or a non-nucleoside reverse transcriptase inhibitor other than Crixivan or Reyataz, it is strongly recommended that you always use a backup method of birth control such as condoms.

Lastly, birth control pills are known to lower blood levels of Agenerase, so these two medications should not be taken together. No studies have been done to determine if there are any potential interactions between HIV treatments and the new methods of birth control including Lunelle shots, Ortho-evra, and the NuvaRING. Although there is not information available yet on possible interactions between Depo shots and HIV treatments, an ongoing study should be giving answers in the near future.

Other relatively common medications known to have interactions with PIs include Zocor, Mevacor, Rifadin, astemizole, terfenadine, Propulsid, midazolam, Halcion, Imitrex, Viagra, and St. John's wort. If there is any question that your blood levels of a certain HIV treatment may be too low from an interaction, your primary care provider can consider checking the blood levels, or performing therapeutic drug monitoring.

HIV Treatments in Pregnancy

In general, pregnant women infected with HIV receive the same treatment as nonpregnant women with HIV. However, the start of treatment may be postponed until after the first trimester (12 weeks), since it is during these early weeks of pregnancy that the unborn baby is most vulnerable to harm from possible medication side effects. But if the mother's CD4 cell count is low and her viral load is very high, it may be deemed more important to start HIV treatments regardless of the age of the fetus. Also, if a woman becomes pregnant while taking HIV treatments, she will risk a rise in her viral load if she temporarily stops taking the medicines.

The one HIV treatment recommended for *all* pregnant women is Retrovir. This drug is recommended even for pregnant women with low viral loads and high CD4 counts. It is an amazing medicine. In a study where Retrovir was given by mouth after 14 weeks gestation, then through the vein during labor, and finally by mouth to the infant, the risk of HIV transmission from the mother to the baby decreased by nearly 70 percent. Because many powerful HIV treatment regimens have been developed since that study was done, today the risk of mother-to-infant transmission of HIV is now only 0 to 2 percent if the mother is taking combination HIV treatment (or at least three HIV treatments).

HIV treatments appear to be reasonably safe to unborn babies and are routinely prescribed during pregnancy. A recent large review of more than 2,000 pregnant women treated with antiretrovirals found HIV treatments were not associated with a premature delivery, low birth weights, or other selected birth complications. Research on HIV treatments in pregnancy is ongoing. In particular, more information is still needed about possible dosing adjustments required during pregnancy. Crixivan has been studied, and its blood levels are known to fall during the last trimester. However, Norvir can be added to the regimen to increase the Crixivan levels (and this also allows the Crixivan to be given only twice daily). Pregnancy is another indication to consider checking blood levels of certain HIV treatments, or therapeutic drug monitoring.

The Food and Drug Administration (FDA) gives a safety rating to every medication it approves, based on the results of extensive testing in both animals and people. All HIV treatments have received an FDA rating of either "class B" or "class C." Class B means that animal studies of the particular medication have not shown any problems in unborn animals. Class C, on the other hand, means that animal studies either have revealed problems with the unborn animals at high doses of the tested medication or that not enough animal data have yet been gathered. Keep in mind that animals and humans do not always react the same way to a given medication.

A registry collects information on the safety of HIV treatments taken in pregnancy. You can encourage your primary care provider to assist with the Antiretroviral Pregnancy Registry by calling 910-251-9087 or 1-800-258-4263. Several long-term studies are also continuing to look at children whose mothers took HIV treatments during pregnancy. These studies watch for any delayed effects on the children from the medications. For further discussion of HIV treatment during pregnancy, see chapter 11.

Do People Ever Stop Treatment?

People have different reasons for wanting to stop taking HIV treatments. For some, the treatments are not working well against the virus. For others, things are going so well that the viral loads have always stayed low and CD4 counts have always stayed high. Some people want to stop because they experience unwanted medication side effects, and some simply get tired of taking so many pills.

Current studies are following what happens to people who stop taking their treatments under certain conditions. This strategy is called *structured treatment interruption*, or STI. There are risks to interrupting therapy, the most worrying of which is that viral loads may rise rapidly after a treatment is interrupted. This may lead to irreversible immune system damage. "Salvage" STI is directed toward patients whose virus has developed many changes and is resistant to most or all drugs. Preliminary studies have shown that "salvage" STI is not a good strategy. Studies are ongoing to address benefits and risks for STI in other groups of patients. The guidelines published in July 2003 do not recommend STI in clinical practice.

What Can We Expect from the Future?

New HIV treatments are approved every year, and new classes of HIV treatments are currently under study. The emphasis is on making powerful treatments more tolerable with fewer side effects. Although a regimen of just one pill a day is not yet available, we now have good regimens consisting of three or more pills that can actually be dosed for once daily.

Fuzeon, or T-20, the first fusion inhibitor, was recently approved. Although persons taking Fuzeon have to deal with taking an injection twice daily, this drug works in people who may have a very resistant virus. Other fusion inhibitors and entry inhibitors are also under study.

KEY POINTS

1. *There are very powerful treatments available that often can control the HIV infection and improve your health.*

2. *Viral load levels usually fall most dramatically to their lowest levels when people start HIV treatments for the first time.*

3. *There are several HIV treatments available and many considerations involved in shaping a treatment plan, including each drug's strength, side effects, dosing schedules, and number of pills per dose.*

4. *A regimen should contain at least three HIV treatments unless you are a pregnant woman taking Retrovir only.*

5. *If you are pregnant and do not need HIV treatment for your own health, you should still take Retrovir to decrease your baby's chances of becoming infected.*

6. *You should be offered HIV treatments for your health if you have symptoms from HIV, if your CD4 cell count is low, or if your viral load level is high.*

7. *You can safely delay HIV treatments if you have no symptoms and you have a high CD4 cell count and a low viral load level.*

8. *It is extremely important to take all doses of all HIV treatments as prescribed. If you do not, your virus may become resistant and the treatments will no longer work.*

9. *Metabolic side effects that may occur with HIV treatments include changes in body shape, increases in blood sugar levels, increases in blood fat levels, and increases in blood acid levels.*

Resources

1. AIDS Treatment News at www.aidsnews.org or FAX 1-415-255-4659 (newsletter on HIV treatments).

2. Pharmaceutical Research and Manufacturers of America (PhRMA) Communication Division at www.phrma.org or call 1-202-835-3400 (PhRMA publishes New Medicines in Development for AIDS, a chart of drugs, tests, and vaccines).

PART THREE

Sexual and Gynecologic Health

Sexual fulfillment is an important part of general health, and while HIV infection leads to changes in sexual practice, it does not mean sacrificing sexual happiness or intimacy. The chapters in this section of the book discuss sexually transmitted diseases and other gynecologic infections as well as HIV.

7

Protecting Yourself and Others

How does a person get HIV?

What is safe sex? What is safer sex?

After having unprotected sex, what can someone do to prevent HIV infection or pregnancy?

How HIV Is Transmitted

When people have HIV, the virus is present in their blood. In women, HIV is also in their vaginal fluid and breast milk; in men, it is present in blood and semen. These are the fluids that can carry the virus from one person to another. There is a much smaller amount of HIV in saliva and tears, and there are no documented cases of HIV being passed from one person to another through either. Anyone infected with HIV can potentially transmit the virus to someone else, regardless of how well the infected person feels or how healthy he or she looks. The virus can be transmitted if infected blood, semen, vaginal fluid, or breast milk enters the body of another person.

While skin is an effective barrier against the virus, it loses its protective qualities wherever it has cuts, sores, or abrasions. Sometimes these breaks in the skin are too tiny to see, and sometimes they are located inside the vagina, rectum, or mouth where they usually go unnoticed if they are not causing pain. The mucous membranes that line the vagina, rectum, and mouth offer some protective barrier if they have no breaks, but even healthy mucous membranes may be less protective than outside skin.

HIV is usually transmitted through unprotected vaginal or rectal sex, through IV drug use (involving needles), through childbirth, and through breastfeeding. Table 7.1 summarizes the risk factors for the sexual transmission of HIV. It is rare for HIV to be transmitted through oral sex, but it is possible. Either the person performing oral sex or the person receiving oral sex can be at risk. Persons who have a break in their mucous membranes from mouth sores are more susceptible, and persons with bleeding gums are infectious.

HIV *cannot* be transmitted through touching, hugging, eating food prepared by someone with HIV or eating after them (eating from the same plate or drinking from the same glass), sharing utensils, swimming in the same pool, or using the same toilet seat. Although there are no established cases of transmission from sharing a toothbrush or razor, it is a bad idea to do this because of the theoretical risk. Finally,

Table 7.1

Risk Factors for Sexual Transmission of HIV to Uninfected Partners

1. An uninfected person with genital sores having unprotected sex with an HIV-infected person, because the HIV can directly enter the bloodstream through the sores.
2. An uninfected person having unprotected sex with an HIV-infected woman during her menstrual period, because there is greater blood exposure.
3. An uninfected person having unprotected sex with an HIV-infected person who has a high viral load.
4. An uninfected woman having unprotected vaginal, anal, or oral sex with an HIV-infected man.
5. An uninfected man having unprotected vaginal, anal, or oral sex with an HIV-infected woman.
6. An uninfected person being the receptive partner of unprotected anal sex with an HIV-infected man.

it is extremely unlikely that someone would get HIV through a blood transfusion because all donated blood is screened for HIV and other blood-borne diseases.

"Safe" Sex and "Safer" Sex

The term "safe sex" refers to sexual activity that poses absolutely no risk of HIV transmission because no one is being exposed to the blood, vaginal secretions, or semen of someone else. Safe sex would include sexual fantasy, self-masturbation, and nonsexual massage. Sexual activity between two HIV-negative people can also be safe with regard to HIV, but only if both partners remain sexually faithful to one another and have no other sexual partners. Of course, sexual abstinence— meaning *no* sex—is also safe.

The term "safer sex" refers to sexual activity that carries a very slight risk for transmission. When used correctly, condoms can be very good at preventing blood, vaginal secretions, or semen from entering a partner's body. However, condoms are not 100 percent effective because they can break or fall off. An estimated 2 to 5 percent of condoms do tear. Water-based lubricants such as KY Jelly can help prevent a condom from breaking and can also increase sexual stimulation. However, be sure to avoid oil-based lubricants like Vaseline, creams, or other oils because these weaken condoms and other latex barriers.

Latex or polyurethane condoms are safer than condoms made from animal skins because animal skin condoms are more porous—they have small holes that may allow transmission of HIV. Other barrier methods of birth control like the diaphragm and the cervical cap do not protect against HIV because they do not cover the entire vagina. Spermicides like nonoxynol-9 offer some protection against pregnancy and against certain sexually transmitted infections like gonorrhea and chlamydia, but they do *not* protect a person from HIV. If used frequently, spermicides may even cause genital sores, which increase the risk for HIV transmission. New types of spermicides that are safer and possibly active against HIV are currently being studied.

There is a slight risk from oral sex if the semen or vaginal secretions get in the mouth. A condom placed over the penis or pieces of latex or plastic placed over the vagina can be used as barriers during oral sex to decrease the risk. It is best not to use a lubricant, because they do not taste very good. You can buy latex dental dams to use during oral sex in dental supply stores.

Fewer than 1 percent of people are truly allergic to latex, which is used in dental dams as well as condoms. If you develop burning or itching after using a latex product, it may be a reaction to the lubricant, the spermicide, or to other materials used in manufacturing. Try changing the brand of latex condoms before assuming you have a latex allergy. If the symptoms persist with a different brand, then try switching to polyurethane condoms. (Because the polyurethane condom called "Avanti" was found to break easily, the manufacturers are now producing a thicker condom with the label "Intended for Latex Sensitive Condom Users Only.") Again, animal skin condoms do not protect against HIV.

Using Condoms Correctly

Condoms only work when they are used correctly. A new condom should be used every time you have sex and should be changed after every ejaculation. Check the condom carefully to make sure it is free of tears before unrolling it onto the erect penis. Be sure to put the condom on before genital contact is made. This is very important, because the drops of liquid that come out of the penis before full ejaculation can contain HIV. If the penis moves from the rectum to the vagina, a new condom should be put on before the penis enters the vagina. If a condom is used twice, it is more likely to break.

To use a condom, place the rolled condom over the tip of the hard penis and unroll it down to the base. Smooth out any air bubbles. If the man is not circumcised, pull the foreskin back before unrolling the condom. After sex, tie a knot in the condom to contain the semen, and throw it away.

The female condom has a flexible ring at both ends. The ring at the closed end is inserted into the vagina to hold the female condom in place. The ring at the open end stays outside the vagina. When you take the condom out of the package, rub it together to spread the lubrication evenly. You can also use additional lubrication. Squeeze the inner ring at the closed end of the pouch and push it up inside the vagina. Make sure that the pouch does not twist. You also need to be careful that the penis does not enter the space between the condom and your vagina. Your partner needs to aim himself straight into the condom.

If you are going to have anal sex, remove the smaller ring to decrease the chance of rectal bleeding. Put the condom over your partner's erect penis. When the penis enters the rectum it will be covered by the condom. Your partner may need to keep his thrusts shallow because the condom is not as long as the rectum. Remove the condom after sex before you stand up. Twist the outer ring and pull the condom out, being careful to keep the semen inside the condom.

Male and female condoms should not be used at the same time.

Unsafe Sex

The term "unsafe sex" refers to sexual activity that involves a high risk of disease transmission because there is direct contact with blood, vaginal secretions, or semen. The rectum, vagina, mouth, nose, and tip of the penis all are very vulnerable to small tears or cuts, which allow the virus a site of entry into the body. Even if a person has no cuts prior to sex, the sexual activity itself can lead to small abrasions. It is important to note that even if both you and your partner have HIV, it is still important to use protection, because one of you may catch a more serious strain of HIV from the other.

Protection after Unsafe Sex

HIV and Other STDs. The best way to protect yourself from unwanted pregnancy, HIV, and other sexually transmitted diseases (STDs) is to avoid unsafe sex. However, there are some after-the-fact measures that may help prevent these outcomes in the event of unsafe sexual contact. They are not 100 percent effective, but they are still worth trying.

The possibility of the recipient (the person being penetrated) catching HIV after having unprotected sex only once is thought to be about 0.1 percent to 3 percent for unprotected anal intercourse and about 0.1 percent to 0.2 percent for unprotected vaginal intercourse. If a condom leaks or breaks, you and your partner should immediately wash your genital areas with soap and water and then quickly apply a spermicide to give some protection against pregnancy and non-HIV infections. Do *not* douche, since this can push the semen higher into the vagina. Also realize that spermicide will not protect against HIV transmission.

Many people wonder if there is a protective benefit from starting on HIV treatments immediately after an episode of unprotected sex. Unfortunately, there is no good information on how well this works. Some clinics do prescribe HIV treatments for people in this situation, but how effective this treatment is depends on the situation and especially on the timing. Ideally, the HIV treatments are started right away and no later than 48 hours after the exposure. The Centers for Disease Control recommends using two HIV medications for four weeks. (See chapter 7 for description of HIV treatments.) There is a national registry at the Centers for Disease Control that is collecting information on this application, which is known as "postexposure prophylaxis." (The CDC registry can be reached at 1-877-488-1737 or on the Internet at www.hivpepppregistry.org.)

In addition to HIV, other sexually transmitted infections can be transmitted during unprotected sex. Chapter 6 discusses hepatitis B and C, and chapter 9 describes other sexually transmitted diseases. If you are not immune to hepatitis B, you should receive the vaccine for protection (see chapter 6 for further information). If you do have unprotected sex, it is extremely important for you to discuss screening and STD prevention with your health care provider—both for your sake and for the sake of your sexual partners.

Pregnancy. Pregnancy is one possible consequence of having unprotected sex. Most women will not get pregnant after only one episode of unprotected sex, but pregnancy is possible after even only one unprotected intercourse, especially if the sex occurs in the middle of the menstrual cycle when the egg is released from the ovary.

The phrase "emergency contraception" refers to taking medications *after* intercourse to prevent pregnancy. Certain estrogen and progesterone preparations can stop the egg from being released and are fairly effective in preventing pregnancy if they are taken within 72 hours after intercourse. Nausea (in up to 50 percent of women) and vomiting (in up to 20 percent) are the main side effects of these medications when taken for emergency contraception. These medicines do not cause abortions because they work largely by blocking ovulation. That means conception cannot happen in the first place. (Abortion refers to interference with an established pregnancy, after the embryo has been implanted in the uterus.)

If you do have an episode of unplanned unprotected sex (such as a broken condom or a rape), you should discuss emergency contraception with a health care provider as soon as possible—ideally within 24 hours. There are two drugs licensed by the Food and Drug Administration for emergency contraception. They are the Yuzpe regimen, also called Preven (ethinyl estradiol and levonorgestrel), and Plan B (levonorgestrel). Plan B is preferable for any woman taking protease inhibitors or non-nucleoside reverse transcriptase inhibitors, which may interact with ethinyl estradiol. In addition, there are less likely to be side effects from Plan B. You can find a provider near you who will prescribe emergency contraception by looking on the Internet at http://ec.princeton.edu/providers.

If you are only using condoms for birth control, you may want to discuss emergency contraception with your primary care provider *before* you need it. Ideally it is a good idea to have the emergency contraception immediately available. If you and your provider agree, fill your prescription for emergency contraception and have it always on hand.

Preventing HIV Transmission at Home

Living and working with HIV-infected people is safe. The virus is *not* transmitted like a common cold. As discussed in the preceding sections, only broken skin or mucous membrane contact with infected bodily fluid can pose a risk of transmission. Gloves, preferably latex, should be worn if there is the possibility of coming into contact with any potentially infectious body fluid. If the gloves are soiled, they should be washed with soap and water and then discarded in a plastic container such as a trash can lined with a plastic bag. If there is any outer skin exposure, wash the area immediately with hot water and soap or other germicide like alcohol. Careful hand washing is very important to prevent the transmission of most infections, not just HIV. Wash your hands under hot running water, vigorously rubbing them together for at least ten seconds with soap or a germicide like alcohol, and then rinse thoroughly.

Fortunately, HIV is easily killed by nearly all chemical disinfectants, including bleach, alcohol (70 percent isopropyl), and hydrogen peroxide. To clean surfaces contaminated by blood or bloody fluids, you can use a 1:10 dilution of a household bleach such as Clorox. (A 1:10 dilution means mixing one part of bleach into nine parts tap water; for example, ½ cup of bleach and 4½ cups of water.) Leave the 1:10 diluted solution on the contaminated surface for ten minutes and then wipe it off. But do not use bleach directly on your skin—not even diluted bleach. If you do get bleach on your skin, or in your eyes or mouth, immediately and thoroughly rinse the affected area with fresh water. Be sure to keep bleach out of the reach of children.

While *undiluted* bleach can leave white spots or holes in clothes and fabric, diluted bleach can usually be used safely on clothes that have been contaminated with blood. If you do have contaminated clothes, presoak these clothes separately with the diluted bleach. Laundry should be washed with detergent using the hot cycle. You do not need to routinely add bleach to every wash; even the diluted bleach may damage some fabrics.

Soiled materials that need to be thrown away, such as sanitary napkins, condoms, or gloves, should be placed in plastic bags for disposal. Liquid waste can be poured into the toilet or sink. The HIV in the sewage is killed through the routine decontamination procedures. Sharp objects like razor blades or needles should be placed either in a "sharps" box that you can get from your health care provider or in a container like a metal coffee can for disposal. It is a good idea to add bleach to the container as an extra precaution, to make sure the HIV is killed.

KEY POINTS

1. *HIV can be transmitted through blood, vaginal fluid, semen, and breast milk if the infected fluid finds its way into another person's body. Transmission can happen through tiny breaks in the skin.*

2. *There are no documented cases of HIV transmission through sweat, tears, or saliva.*

3. *The only guaranteed protection from HIV transmission is total avoidance of sex (called sexual abstinence) or choosing only "safe sex" activities like fantasy, self-masturbation, nonsexual massage, and sex with your partner if you are only sexually active with each other and no one else (monogamous sex) and neither of you is HIV-infected.*

4. *"Safer sex" is sex that carries a very slight risk for transmission, such as sex with condoms.*

5. *The possibility of becoming infected with HIV after having sex only once is thought to be about 0.1 to 3 percent for unprotected receptive anal intercourse and 0.1 to 0.2 percent for unprotected receptive vaginal intercourse.*

6. *Some clinics will prescribe prophylactic HIV treatments (to prevent HIV transmission) after an episode of unprotected sex, depending on the situation and timing. The HIV treatments should be started within 48 hours after the exposure.*

7. *Certain estrogen and progesterone preparations are fairly effective in preventing pregnancy if taken within 72 hours after unprotected sex.*

8

Gynecologic Infections and Sexually Transmitted Diseases

What causes a vaginal discharge?

What causes vaginal or pelvic infections and how are they treated?

What causes genital sores and how are they treated?

In this chapter we describe the common infections and diseases of the female reproductive organs. A woman who has any of the symptoms of infection or disease described in this chapter should see her health care provider for advice and treatment.

Vaginal Discharge

Any healthy woman may have vaginal discharge, but not all vaginal discharge is healthy. Abnormal discharge may indicate the woman has an infection, and infection may require treatment. This chapter will help you recognize the signs and symptoms of many gynecologic infections that are common medical problems in all women, whether they have HIV or not. Most cases of abnormal vaginal discharge are caused by three different types of infections: bacterial vaginosis, vaginal yeast,

Table 8.1
Vaginal Infections

Infection	Main symptom	Sexually transmitted?
Bacterial vaginosis	fishy odor, white or gray vaginal discharge	no
Vaginal yeast infection	vaginal itching, white vaginal discharge	no
Trichomonas vaginitis	heavy yellow or greenish vaginal discharge, spotting	yes

and trichomoniasis. Table 8.1 summarizes the symptoms of these three infections.

Bacterial Vaginosis

Bacterial vaginosis (BV) is one of the most common causes of abnormal vaginal discharge. It is harder for women with HIV to clear a BV infection than for women without HIV. The lower a woman's CD4 count, the more likely it is that she will have trouble clearing a BV infection. The first thing most women notice about BV is not the discharge but rather a strong, fishy-smelling vaginal odor. The thick discharge of a BV infection is generally described as either gray or white in color. BV is thought to result from an overgrowth of certain bacteria that normally live in the vagina in smaller numbers. BV is *not* considered a sexually transmitted infection. It is diagnosed by your primary care provider or gynecologist looking at a swab of vaginal discharge under the microscope. The acidity of the discharge, its appearance, and its smell assist in making the diagnosis.

For some women, BV in pregnancy may be related to premature delivery. Treating BV in women who have had a history of premature delivery has been shown in some studies to decrease the chance of another premature delivery. Other studies have compared the rates of post-delivery infections among women who delivered their babies by cesarean section. These studies found that women with BV had five times the rate of post-delivery infections as women without BV. Because of these findings, your primary care provider or obstetrician may want to screen you for BV if you are pregnant, but routine screening of every pregnant woman is not recommended by experts.

Treatment for BV infection involves either pills or a topical cream or gel applied to the vagina. Usually the oral medication Flagyl (metronidazole) is prescribed. The topical treatments include Cleocin (clindamycin) cream and Flagyl (metronidazole) gel. A course of oral Flagyl is very inexpensive, costing less than five dollars. In contrast, the cream and gel treatments cost over $25. If you use Flagyl, you should not drink alcohol during treatment and for 24 hours after treatment ends, because drinking alcohol while on Flagyl will make you sick. Cleocin cream is oil-based and might weaken latex condoms and diaphragms, so it's a good idea to avoid sex while using Cleocin. Unfortunately, as many as 30 percent of women treated for BV find that their symptoms return again within one month.

Vaginal Yeast

If you have a vaginal yeast infection, you may have symptoms of vaginal itching, burning, and soreness. Yeast infections are common and often appear after a woman has taken a course of antibiotics for some other reason. They are not sexually transmitted. The diagnosis is made based on the symptoms as well as on the appearance of the discharge (which is often compared to cottage cheese); diagnosis can be confirmed by your primary care provider or gynecologist examining the discharge under a microscope.

Yeast infections are common in women with low CD4 counts. While not all women with HIV get vaginal yeast infections, some struggle with them constantly unless they take anti-yeast medication all the time. For some women the infection never completely clears.

To treat yeast infections, it is best first to try topical creams or lozenges inserted into the vagina. These treatments range in price from about $10 to $25. Although many women prefer taking a pill, Diflucan (fluconazole), instead of using a cream, it is better to reserve the pill for situations where the cream does not work. Generally women with HIV require more than one dose of Diflucan. The problem with taking Diflucan constantly is that the yeast can become resistant to it, making the medicine useless. However, it does appear to be safe to take Diflucan just once a week to *prevent* vaginal yeast infections. Miconazole (Monistat) 100 mg vaginal cream or Terezol vaginal cream are the treatments of choice during pregnancy. Treatments for vaginal yeast infections are available both over-the-counter (without a prescription) and with a prescription (usually stronger medications).

If you seem to get a yeast infection any time you take antibiotics, you should either begin using an over-the-counter treatment as soon as you begin taking antibiotics or let your primary care provider know about the problem so you can get a prescription for an anti-yeast medication whenever you need to take antibiotics.

Trichomoniasis

Unlike bacterial vaginosis and vaginal yeast, trichomoniasis *is* sexually transmitted. This infection may cause no symptoms at all, or it may cause a bothersome heavy discharge that may be greenish or yellow. Some women have itching and soreness. Your primary care provider will diagnose this infection from a Pap smear result or by using a microscope to see active trichomonads. Because this infection is transmitted through sex, it is important that your partner also be treated. Otherwise, you will catch the infection again from your partner. The only treatment for trichomoniasis is Flagyl (metronidazole) taken by mouth, which costs less than five dollars. Topical treatment with Flagyl cream is not effective for trichomoniasis.

Pelvic Infections

Women's reproductive anatomy is capable of tremendous change. The uterus, a thick muscle normally the size of a closed fist or pear, can expand in pregnancy to envelop a big baby—or even more than one baby!

Before considering the problems that can afflict the female pelvis, it is worth taking a minute to appreciate the power and resilience of the organs it contains. The uterus, also called the womb, sits at the top of the vagina. Every month the uterus sheds its lining through the vagina in a monthly period. The cervix is a small ring of tissue that connects the top of the vagina to the uterus. The cervix can expand to 10 centimeters wide during childbirth. Pap smear samples are taken from the cervix, and an infection of the cervix is called cervicitis. (Not all cervical infections cause symptoms, so women often have an infection without realizing it. The most common causes of cervicitis in women are gonorrhea and chlamydia. Gonorrhea and chlamydia are bacteria that can be transmitted through sex.)

Two fallopian tubes lead from the uterus to the space very near the ovaries on either side of the body. Because the tubes are open on both ends, the female pelvis is really connected to the outside world. It is not sealed off. This means that bacteria entering the vagina can make their way up the vagina, through the cervix, across the uterus, down the fallopian tubes, and into the pelvis. Part of the value of normal vaginal discharge is to continually wash the system, sweeping germs out of the body.

Pelvic inflammatory disease, commonly known as PID, occurs when the uterus and tubes become infected. Unlike cervicitis, which may have no symptoms, PID will always make a woman feel sick. She may have stomach or pelvic pain, nausea, vomiting, abnormal vaginal discharge, fever, and chills. These symptoms can also result from other dangerous medical or obstetrical problems such as a kidney infection, appendicitis, or ectopic pregnancy (a medical emergency that occurs when the embryo has implanted outside the uterus, usually in one of the fallopian tubes). If you have these symptoms, seek medical care immediately.

Women with severe symptoms from PID may require surgery to drain the infection. Because of the possible consequences of PID, which include the risk of permanent tube scarring and infertility, early treatment with strong antibiotics is important. While some women may be treated successfully as outpatients, others require hospitalization to receive antibiotics through a vein if they have trouble taking the medications or if they do not rapidly improve.

PID can cause long-term problems such as chronic pelvic pain, difficulty becoming pregnant, and a tendency toward ectopic pregnancies. After one episode of PID, a woman's risk of ectopic pregnancy increases sevenfold compared with the risk for women who have no history of PID. If a woman has had three or more episodes of PID, she has a 50 percent chance of being unable to get pregnant. Fifteen to 20 percent of women with PID have complications requiring surgery. Complications include pockets of infection called "abscesses" and scar tissue that may cause pain and must be surgically removed.

Several studies performed in the United States and Africa have compared the symptoms of PID in women with and without HIV. These studies have shown that women with HIV have a lower white blood cell count (these are the cells that fight bacterial infections) and are more likely to require surgery to clear the infection. They are also more likely to continue to have fevers even after treatment. The types of bacteria causing PID appear to be similar in women with and without HIV. As with cervicitis, the most common bacteria responsible for PID are gonorrhea and chlamydia, which are both sexually transmitted and which often travel together.

It is easy to screen for both gonorrhea and chlamydia using simple urine tests. Women are also routinely screened for these two infections during their regular pelvic exams, with a test based on the cervical swab. If you are sexually active, you can decrease your risk for PID by having your primary care provider check you every six months for gonorrhea and chlamydia. Up to 40 percent of women with cervicitis who do not receive treatment for these two common infections develop PID, so it is a very good idea to get regular screening—especially because treatment is so simple and avoids potentially serious complications.

The most frequently used treatment for chlamydia is one dose of the antibiotic Zithromax (azithromycin), which costs about $30. However, Vibramycin (doxycycline), erythromycin, and Floxin (ofloxacin) are also effective. A seven-day course of Vibramycin usually costs less than five dollars. There are several treatments for gonorrhea, including pills such as Suprax (cefixime), Cipro (ciprofloxacin), and Floxin (ofloxacin). One dose of Rocephin (cephtriaxone) can also be given, administered as an injection into a muscle. The cost of the pills ranges from less than $5 to over $15. Vibramycin and Floxin should not be given to pregnant women, and Floxin should not be used in girls younger than 18 years of age. Because gonorrhea and chlamydia are both sexually transmitted, the sexual partners of anyone diagnosed with these infections also need to receive treatment.

Genital Ulcers (Sores)

The most likely cause for genital sores in the United States is a rampant viral infection called herpes simplex virus, or HSV-2. About one in five Americans over the age of 12 has been infected with HSV-2 (genital herpes), but less than 20 percent of them are *aware* of having been infected. Blood test results have diagnosed HSV-2 in at least 45 million people in the United States, and the proportion of infected people has increased about 30 percent in the last twenty years. A second frequent cause of genital sores is syphilis, and a third infection, called chancroid, is uncommon in the United States and very infrequent among women. Other rare infections can cause genital sores in HIV-infected women with low CD4 cell counts. HIV itself can do this, as can a virus called CMV (cytomegalovirus). The following paragraphs discuss each of these infections in turn, and table 8.2 summarizes the causes of genital sores.

Herpes Simplex Virus

The sores of HSV-2 erupt and then subside. When sores are present, a person is said to be having a "flare." The infection is most contagious to others during a flare, and symptoms are most unpleasant. In between flares, a person may feel fine, but during a flare symptoms typically include genital pain, burning, itching, or stinging. These uncomfortable symptoms often occur one to four days before the genital sores appear. At first, the sores caused by HSV-2 look like groups of small blisters, and they hurt. These little blisters develop into sores over the course of a few days. In women with HIV, the sores can become very

Table 8.2
Infectious Causes of Genital Sores

Cause	Main symptom	CD4 relationship	Sexually transmitted?
Common			
HSV-2	recurrent painful blisters or sores	sores worse with low CD4	yes
Syphilis	one or few sores, rash (often on hands and feet)	no influence on sores	yes
Rare			
CMV	deep, painful sores	usually low CD4	*
HIV	deep, painful sores	usually low CD4	*
Chancroid	one or few painful sores	no information	yes

Note: HSV-2 = genital herpes simplex virus. CMV = cytomegalovirus
* CMV and HIV are transmitted sexually, but the sores are not. The genital sores have only been described in women.

deep and wide, especially among women with low CD4 cell counts. HSV-2 can be controlled but not yet cured.

Generally the first outbreak of HSV-2 is the most severe, and it can leave a person feeling very sick, with swollen lymph nodes. Repeat episodes of HSV-2 sores are usually not as bad as the initial outbreak, and they heal more rapidly. Stress and the start of the menstrual period may trigger a flare. To determine whether a genital sore is from HSV-2, the sore must be swabbed to obtain a culture for laboratory testing. Another way to check for HSV-2 is by looking for the virus's DNA with a polymerase chain reaction (PCR) test. It is not uncommon to have a negative culture result yet still be infected with HSV-2. So, depending on how the sores look, your provider may still suggest treating you for this infection even if you have a negative result.

HSV-2 can be sexually transmitted or transmitted by skin-to-skin contact. If you touch an open sore, the virus can be carried by your skin to other places on your body, such as the eye. To prevent transmission from a pregnant woman to her baby, women with HSV-2 are often advised to have cesarean sections rather than to risk vaginal delivery.

The goal of HSV-2 treatment is to prevent symptom outbreaks, because we do not yet have a way to cure the disease altogether. Fortunately, pills can be very effective in controlling the virus (they work better than topical treatments). The three pills available to treat the infection are Zovirax (acyclovir), Famvir (famciclovir), and Valtrex (valcyclovir). The costs of these treatments range from approximately $20 to $100. Staying on treatment decreases the chance of flares by 75 percent. Although HSV-2 is sexually transmitted, partners are not treated because the treatment does not cure the disease but only decreases the symptoms.

The only one of these treatments that has been carefully studied in pregnancy is Zovirax, and so far it seems to be safe. Zovirax treatment is recommended during pregnancy for initial outbreaks and also in the last trimester for women who have had frequent outbreaks, with the goal of preventing a flare at the time of delivery. Valtrex and Famvir have not been adequately studied during pregnancy. With help from the Centers for Disease Control, the makers of Zovirax and Valtrex maintain a registry to review the use of these medications during pregnancy. (The registry's telephone number is 800-722-9292, extension 38465. Sharing your experience in taking these medications with the registry will help in the study of the effects of taking these medications during pregnancy.)

Syphilis

Syphilis is a sexually transmitted disease that can do terrible harm to the body if it goes untreated—but that fortunately is very easy to diagnose and treat. The genital sores associated with syphilis usually are not painful, and even without treatment the sores will get better in three to eight weeks. But this does *not* mean the infection is gone.

Among untreated people, about half have syphilis spread throughout the body. When this happens, a rash almost always follows, along with fever, sore throat, headache, swollen lymph nodes, hair loss, and an inflamed liver. Pregnant women are routinely screened for syphilis because the infection can pass from mother to baby.

Syphilis is diagnosed by using a special microscope called a *dark field microscope* to examine a swab of discharge taken from a sore. The other usual method of diagnosis is a blood test (VDRL, ART, or RPR), but these blood tests can sometimes be falsely positive—meaning that the test will indicate syphilis when in fact there is no syphilis. Because this problem is familiar to health care providers, a second test is ordered to confirm any positive blood test result. If your initial blood test is positive, it might remain positive for the rest of your life. Therefore, if you have been diagnosed with syphilis at some time in the past, don't be surprised if every clinic you go to wants to treat you again for syphilis because of your positive blood test. You can also have a false negative blood test if your body has not yet had time to make the antibodies, so your primary care provider may wish to repeat the test at a later date.

Penicillin cures syphilis. The medicine is best administered as a series of one to three shots into the muscle. The number of recommended shots depends on how long a person has been infected with syphilis. Each shot costs about $35. Because syphilis is sexually transmitted, the sexual partners of anyone diagnosed with the disease should also receive penicillin. During pregnancy, penicillin is the only recommended treatment. If a pregnant woman is allergic to penicillin, her obstetrician may recommend hospitalization to "desensitize" her to this highly effective treatment. Desensitization involves first giving a very small dose of penicillin under careful observation, and then, when there is no severe reaction, gradually increasing the dose as the body grows accustomed to the drug.

CMV and HIV

Less common causes of genital sores include HIV and the virus called *cytomegalovirus*, or CMV. If test results for HSV-2 and syphilis come back negative for a person with genital sores, then health care providers will often want to obtain a biopsy sample to look for CMV or order special cultures to look for chancroid (which is not a common infection in the United States). A biopsy can be performed in an outpatient clinic and involves taking a small piece of tissue for testing. If the biopsy reveals the presence of CMV, then anti-CMV treatments can be given through the vein and will often improve symptoms. These treatments include Cytovene (ganciclovir), Vistide (cidofovir), and Foscavir (foscarnet).

If the biopsy does *not* reveal CMV and if the cultures are negative, then HIV itself may be causing the sores. Generally sores caused by HIV are severe and painful. However, they may improve if you start on HIV treatment. Other therapies, such as steroids and thalidomide, have also been shown to help. Be aware that thalidomide causes very severe birth defects, and for this reason all sexually active women who are capable of becoming pregnant and are prescribed thalidomide must use *at least two forms of birth control*, for example, a hormonal birth control method and condoms.

KEY POINTS

1. *Abnormal vaginal discharge can result from vaginal, cervical, or pelvic infection as well as from genital sores.*

2. *Vaginal infections include bacterial vaginosis, yeast infections, and trichomoniasis—all of which are easily treated.*

3. *Cervical and pelvic infections are usually caused by chlamydia or gonorrhea, which are also easily treated.*

4. *Trichomoniasis, chlamydia, and gonorrhea are all transmitted through sexual contact, and partners should also be treated. You should be checked for these infections if you are sexually active.*

5. *The most common causes of genital sores among HIV-infected women are herpes simplex virus-2 and syphilis. Both are sexually transmitted.*

9

Human Papillomavirus Infections,
Genital Warts, and Abnormal Pap Smears

---

*What is human papillomavirus and what problems
can it cause?*

What treatments are available for genital warts?

How often should Pap smears be done?

*Do women with abnormal Pap smears need to
be treated?*

*What special risks do women with HIV have for
human papillomavirus infections, genital warts, or
abnormal Pap smears?*

Human Papillomavirus Infections

Human papillomavirus (HPV) is a very common infection of the genitals and cervix. It can be transmitted through sex or by skin-to-skin
contact. It may be a lifelong infection or it may clear from the body.
HPV causes no symptoms in many women, but in other women it
causes genital warts and abnormal Pap smear results. The Pap smear
(named for George Papanicolaou, who developed the test) is a painless

test for cervical cancer. To do a Pap smear, the primary care provider or gynecologist collects a thin layer of cells from the cervix, using a brush or swab. These cells are then evaluated under the microscope by a pathologist. (Table 9.1 describes various Pap smear results; see below for details on abnormal Pap results.)

HPV has many strains, some more serious than others. The high-risk strains are associated with cancer of the cervix. These particular strains are numbered 16, 18, 31, and 35. women with HIV and low CD4 counts or high viral loads are more likely to be infected with HPV and to have abnormal Pap smears. Women with a low CD4 cell count may be less likely to fight off the infection or clear it from their bodies.

A woman who has genital warts usually is infected with HPV. Pap

Table 9.1
Pap Smear Results: What Do They Mean?

Result	What it means
Normal	No pathology found
Inflammatory atypia	Atypical cells probably caused by a vaginal or cervical infection
Atypical squamous cells of undetermined significance (ASCUS)	Atypical cells often caused by an HPV infection
HPV effects	Abnormal findings from HPV infection
Mild dysplasia*	Mild precancer findings
Moderate dysplasia*	Moderate precancer findings
Severe dysplasia*	Severe precancer findings
Carcinoma in situ	Cancerlike changes that are microscopic (can only be detected with the microscope)
Invasive carcinoma	Cancer that has invaded into the cervix or spread beyond the cervix

* Other medical terms that refer to dysplasia or precancer findings of the cervix include *cervical intraepithelial neoplasia* (or *CIN*) and *squamous intraepithelial lesions* (or *SIL*). *CIN1* or *low-grade SIL* refer to mild precancer findings; *CIN2* or *high-grade SIL* refer to moderate precancer findings; and *CIN3* refers to carcinoma in situ (noninvasive cancer).

smear results can reveal the presence of HPV even in women who have no visible genital warts. A Pap smear looks for typical changes to cells that HPV can cause. There are other tests available that will check for specific HPV types, but these tests are not routinely used because their results do not make a difference in treatment planning. Recommendations for treatment are based either on the presence of warts or on the finding of precancerous or cancerous cells in the Pap smear. Not everyone with HPV infection needs to be treated.

Treatment for Genital Warts

It can be difficult to predict whether genital warts will resolve on their own, persist without changing, or get worse. Even with treatment, the warts often return. They typically appear on the vagina, cervix, and rectum. Treatments include topical medications and various office procedures. Two prescribed topical treatments that a woman can do at home are Condylox (podofilox) 0.5% solution or gel (take up to 4 cycles) and Aldara (imiquimod) 5% cream (take for up to 16 weeks). These treatments are expensive, ranging from approximately $70 to over $100. Acids can be applied to warts in the office by your primary care provider or gynecologist. Other outpatient clinic treatments include freezing the warts (cryotherapy) or burning them with a small laser. If you are pregnant, not all options are recommended, and your obstetrician will work with you to develop the best treatment plan. Warts often enlarge with pregnancy and then shrink after delivery.

How Often Should Women Have Pap Smears?

Women with HIV are two to three times more likely than HIV-negative women to be infected with HPV. Abnormal Pap smear results are therefore very common in women with HIV: up to 40 percent of women with HIV have abnormal results on their Pap smear, some of which may be caused by HPV.

Because of this increased risk for abnormal Pap results, the Centers for Disease Control recommends that every woman have a Pap smear

Table 9.2

Recommended Follow-up for Pap Smears

Pap smear result	Follow-up
Normal	Yearly Pap smears*
Inflammatory atypia	Treat any infections and repeat Pap smear in 3 months; if repeat Pap smears show atypia, then colposcopy
ASCUS, HPV effects, any dysplasia, and cancer	Colposcopy**

* A second Pap smear should be done 6 months after the first (baseline) Pap smear. If results of both smears are normal, then yearly examinations are recommended.

** Generally a Pap smear or colposcopy is done every 3 to 6 months for follow-up if findings are ASCUS, HPV effects, or mild dysplasia. Some providers may wish first to repeat the Pap smear for a woman with ASCUS, particularly if the woman also has a vaginal or cervical infection. Women with recurrent ASCUS should have colposcopy, however. Treatment is generally recommended if a cervical biopsy shows moderate or severe dysplasia or cancer.

done when she is first diagnosed with HIV. If the results come back normal, then a second Pap smear should be done in six months. If that too is normal, then Pap smears are recommended once a year thereafter. However, if results are not normal, then women are followed more closely and treatment may be needed.

Table 9.2 summarizes the recommended frequency for Pap smears based on the findings, and refers to a procedure called *colposcopy*, which is described in the following section. Note that these recommendations remain the same for all women who have had hysterectomies.

Abnormal Pap Smears, Colposcopy, and Treatment

The Pap smear allows a pathologist to get a close look at individual cells from the cervix. Changes from normal take different forms and have different names. The most common abnormal Pap smear result is reported as "atypical squamous cells of undetermined significance," or

"ASCUS." Other common results include "HPV effects" and "mild dysplasia" (which is also termed "precancerous," even though precancer cells do not necessarily turn into cancer). It is worth emphasizing that these findings are very common and that most women with dysplasia do not develop cancer. Close follow-up with repeat Pap smears is necessary, however, and a colposcopy procedure is often recommended. While these common cervical cell changes sometimes clear on their own and even return to normal, the changes may get worse and potentially lead to cancer.

What is colposcopy? The "colposcope" is basically a powerful magnifying glass with a light. Using this instrument, your provider can carefully examine the cervix to look for any areas that appear abnormal. If any part of the cervix appears abnormal, the provider can then take a biopsy (a small tissue sample) to check for cancer. This examination ensures that any cell biopsy will be taken from a part of the cervix most likely to have an abnormality, rather than from a healthy part of the cervix. If your Pap smear result is abnormal, you should have a colposcopy to be sure that you do not have cancer. The procedure is generally done in an outpatient clinic and takes about twenty minutes. Most women experience only mild discomfort, but a woman may experience mild, menstrual-like cramps after the procedure if a cervical biopsy is taken.

Some studies have shown that women with HIV are more likely to clear HPV infection and improve their abnormal Pap smear results when they begin taking HIV treatments, possibly because the treatments strengthen the immune system to fight HPV. Studies evaluating the relationships between CD4 cell counts, viral loads, HIV treatments, HPV infections, and Pap smear results are currently ongoing.

If the results of a cervical biopsy indicate moderate or severe dysplasia, then treatment is generally recommended. The goal of treatment is to get rid of the abnormal cervical cells. Several different procedures can accomplish this. The "loop electrosurgical excision procedure"—or "LEEP"—involves burning the cells. It is an outpatient procedure that sounds worse than it is. Most women do not have trouble with the LEEP. Possible complications from a LEEP include bleeding (which occurs in less than 2 percent of women) and "cervical stenosis," which means that the cervical opening becomes smaller as the cervix heals after LEEP. (Cervical stenosis occurs in 1 percent of women.)

A second procedure, called "cone excision," involves cutting the cells out of the body, and requires a short hospital stay, generally just one day. Hysterectomy, which is a more substantial surgery to remove the entire uterus and cervix, is generally recommended only when a woman has cervical cancer or when there are other reasons for her to have a hysterectomy.

If you have had moderate to severe cervical dysplasia, you have a 40 percent to 60 percent chance of being diagnosed again with this same finding, even after treatment. Recurrent dysplasia requiring treatment occurs more often in women with low CD4 cell counts. However, there is a home treatment that decreases the chances of recurrence. When a vaginal suppository of 5-FU (5-fluorouracil) cream is applied to the cervix twice weekly for six months, the likelihood of recurrence falls to only 8 percent. Some gynecologists are reluctant to prescribe 5-FU because it has the possible side effect of vaginal irritation; it should not be used in pregnancy.

Cervical Cancer

Cervical cancer became an AIDS-defining condition in 1993. But even though abnormal Pap smears are common among women with HIV, cervical cancer is not. Usually women with cervical cancer have a CD4 cell count below 200. The treatment of cervical cancer among women with HIV does not differ from the treatment recommended for HIV-negative women, but starting HIV treatment may strengthen the immune system to help fight the cancer.

KEY POINTS

1. Infection with human papillomavirus (HPV) can cause genital warts and changes in the cervix. The cervix may develop precancerous changes or cancer.

2. HIV infection increases the risk for HPV infections, genital warts, and abnormal Pap smear results.

3. When a woman is first diagnosed with HIV, she should have a Pap smear. The recommended frequency of repeat Pap smears will depend on the results.

4. Women with HIV who receive abnormal Pap smear results should have a colposcopy and possibly a biopsy done to look for cervical cancer.

5. Recommendations for treatment following an abnormal Pap smear result depend on the result.

PART FOUR

Reproduction

Deciding whether or not to have a baby can be difficult in the best of circumstances, but living with HIV makes this decision even more complicated. The following chapters describe options for birth control, the nature of the menstrual life cycle, and how HIV can change the experience of pregnancy.

10

Considering Pregnancy and Birth Control

What factors should partners discuss when considering pregnancy and birth control?

If a couple wants to have children and only one partner has HIV, are there ways to decrease the risk of HIV transmission to the uninfected partner?

What influences a woman's chances of becoming pregnant?

What can a couple do if they are having problems becoming pregnant?

What factors increase the risk of complications during pregnancy?

What are the risks and benefits of different reversible birth control options?

How do hormonal birth control methods interact with HIV treatments?

Considering Pregnancy

The decision to become pregnant is one of the most important decisions a woman will ever make. Becoming pregnant should not be left to chance, and a decision to become pregnant should be made after careful thought and discussion with your partner. This holds true for any woman, but for women with HIV, there are additional considerations to weigh. Having HIV does not necessarily mean that you cannot get pregnant, nor does it mean that you should not. If you are sexually active and of childbearing age, you probably have the ability to conceive. However, every woman with HIV should be aware of the potential risks that this chronic disease poses. For a woman with HIV, the decision to become pregnant should only be made after careful consideration of what is known about how HIV may affect mother and child. Some topics that you may wish to discuss with your primary care provider or obstetrician before you become pregnant are:

- The effects of HIV on pregnancy and on the unborn baby
- The effects that other medical conditions may have on your pregnancy and unborn baby
- The effect of pregnancy on your health
- The risk of passing HIV to your unborn baby and how to decrease that risk
- The effects of HIV treatments on the unborn baby
- The effects of other prescribed medications on pregnancy or on the unborn baby
- The effects of alcohol or recreational drug use on pregnancy and on the unborn baby
- Your health and the health of your partner over the next 18 years

One of the biggest concerns that women with HIV have about becoming pregnant is whether their babies will be born with HIV. There are no guarantees, but it has been well established that your chances of transmitting the HIV infection to your baby are influenced by how well your own HIV infection is controlled. If you have a high viral load and a low CD4 count, the risk of transmission is much higher than if you have a low viral load and a high CD4 count. Certain medical conditions, such as hepatitis C, can increase the risk of HIV transmission to the baby and diseases such as diabetes or epilepsy can increase the risk of pregnancy complications.

Because medicines can cross from the mother's blood into the baby's blood, you also need to think about the possible influence of any medications you take regularly. Many medications are not recommended during pregnancy. Several pain medications should not be taken during pregnancy, for example. Non-steroidal anti-inflammatory drugs (NSAIDs) such as Motrin or Naprosyn can affect the baby's development and are not advised in pregnancy. In addition, your baby can become addicted to opioids or narcotics if you take these drugs (see chapter 14). Other medications that are prescribed for chronic medical or psychiatric conditions can also be dangerous to the unborn baby. Sometimes your provider can substitute a safer alternative, but not always. It is important to review all of your medications with your primary care provider before you become pregnant because many drugs are most harmful to the fetus during the first eight weeks of pregnancy. It is difficult but necessary to consider which medicines are absolutely required for your own health and well-being and which you might be able to do without. *No changes in medications should be made without first talking to your primary care provider,* however, even if you learn you are pregnant. The risk of stopping certain medications may be more dangerous to your unborn baby than the medication exposure.

If you are on HIV treatments now and are considering becoming pregnant, it is a good idea to talk with your primary care provider about each of your specific medicines. Although most HIV treatments are considered to be reasonably safe during pregnancy, some are known to cause problems. For example, pregnant women should not take Sustiva, the liquid solution of Agenerase, or Hydrea. It is better to have your treatment regimen adjusted *before* you conceive a baby because many drugs are most harmful during the first eight weeks of pregnancy.

Most HIV treatments have not been available for very long. We do not yet know if the future will reveal long-term effects on babies who were exposed to them. However, long-term studies are being done right now to monitor children whose mothers took HIV treatment while pregnant, so in several years we will have much more information about the long-term safety of these treatments. Primary care providers can report any experience with HIV treatments used in pregnant women to the Antiretroviral Pregnancy Registry. Although there has not been enough information to report on the safety of most treatments, the experience with Viracept, one of the most commonly used treatments in pregnancy, was recently described. Among 301 women who took Viracept during their first trimester, there was no increase in birth defects over what would be expected in the general population.

Pregnancy requires a certain amount of strength, and maintaining a healthy weight is very important. Your health care provider can help you plan a nutritious diet. Being underweight or overweight can increase the chances of complications. Pregnant women need to consume many more calories than do nonpregnant women. Growing babies automatically take the nutrition they need from their mother's blood, and without an adequate diet the mother's needs will go unmet. She will become weak, tired, and possibly sick. If a nonpregnant woman is already having trouble maintaining her own weight, she will have a much harder time doing so once a baby is growing inside. Chronic health problems such as diarrhea or nausea can interfere with the pregnant woman's ability to take in and absorb sufficient calories.

As a woman ages, it becomes more difficult for her to become pregnant. Women older than 35 years have increasing difficulty becoming pregnant, and when they do become pregnant, their babies have a higher chance of developmental problems like Down's syndrome. Compared to younger women, women over 35 also have approximately twice the risk for diabetes, high blood pressure, and vaginal bleeding during pregnancy.

When Only One of You Has HIV

A couple in which only one of the partners has been infected with HIV is called a "discordant" couple. Many discordant couples want to have children but do not want to transmit the HIV from one parent to the other or to the baby. What can you do if you wish to have a baby with someone, and one of you has HIV? One strategy that will decrease the chances of HIV transmission is for the infected person to decrease his or her viral load to nondetectable levels by taking HIV treatments. Other strategies depend on which partner has HIV.

When the Woman Has HIV

If the woman has HIV and the man does not, his sperm can be inserted into the vagina at home using a simple syringe (without a needle). This is called the "turkey baster" method. You can obtain the syringe from your primary care provider or purchase one at the drug store. Buy the syringe with the plunger, not the bulb end. The man ejaculates into a sterile cup, and then the semen is drawn into the syringe. Take the syringe and draw up all the semen. Be sure to tap out any air bubbles. You can do this by slowly rotating the syringe until the opening is facing up. Tap the air bubbles to the top and then gently push the plunger just enough to push out the air.

Get into a comfortable position to insert the syringe into the vagina. Slowly insert the syringe and gently push out the semen. The goal is to coat the outside of your cervix. Once the semen has been inserted into the vagina, the sperm will have a better chance of reaching the egg if the woman uses gravity to help. One position for achieving this goal is to get on your hands and knees with your shoulders down and your hips up.

Insemination can also be performed in a fertility clinic using a small tube that inserts the sperm directly into the cervix. Regardless of whether insemination is done at home or in the clinic, timing is important for success. Insemination should take place either during ovulation or just prior to ovulation. Ovulation occurs in the middle of the menstrual cycle (generally 14 days after your period begins). See below for how to monitor your "basal temperature" to determine more precisely when ovulation occurs for you.

When the Man Has HIV

If the man has HIV and the woman does not, it becomes more difficult to achieve pregnancy while avoiding HIV transmission. But there are a few strategies to try. We know that the amount of HIV in the semen correlates with the amount of HIV in the blood, so one of the best strategies to prevent transmission is for the male partner with HIV to reduce his viral load to undetectable levels with HIV treatment. While it is still possible for there to be HIV in the genital tract even when the blood levels of HIV are too low to be detected, usually the blood viral load is a good indicator of the viral load in the semen.

Another strategy is sperm washing, which involves separating the sperm from the other fluid components in semen. Only the sperm are needed to conceive a baby, and at this time, although research continues on this question, it is thought that HIV probably does not attach to or infect the sperm. If the sperm are washed free of other liquids in the ejaculated semen that do contain HIV, the risk of potential transmission is probably decreased. The washed sperm specimen can be checked for HIV prior to insemination. At one European center that provides this service, the chances of the specimen still having detectable HIV after washing was 6 percent. Infected specimens are not used for insemination. Sperm washing has been controversial in the United States, and few centers have offered this service. A recent publication from the New Jersey Medical School outlined their criteria for offering this service (see table 10.1). Two additional centers that have offered sperm washing are Columbia University in New York (212-305-4665) and the Assisted Reproduction Foundation in Boston (718-665-0750). We hope more centers will follow their lead and offer this service.

Regardless of the precautions you take, there is still a slight risk for transmission. Ideally your primary care provider or gynecologist will perform a few tests to maximize the chance of a pregnancy occurring so that the man or woman has the least possible exposure to HIV. These tests include sperm analysis and the woman's reproductive hormone levels. Sexual intercourse or insemination should be timed to occur just

Table 10.1

Criteria and Recommendations for Use of Assisted Reproductive Technologies among HIV-Infected Men and Women at New Jersey Medical School in Newark

1. Disclosure of HIV between partners
2. Counseling before trying to become pregnant
3. Informed consent (must explain risks, benefits, alternatives)
4. No infections or cancers described in chapter 4
5. CD4 cell count more than 350 cells/mm^3 and a viral load less than 50,000
6. Persons receiving HIV treatments must have the following
   - a nondetectable viral load
   - not taking any medications that could seriously harm the baby
   - able to take their HIV treatments without problems
   - stable on HIV treatments for at least one year
7. Semen samples checked for HIV before insemination (only negative samples used)
8. Retrovir during labor
9. Follow-up of child (strongly recommended)
10. HIV-infected women must have normal results on their Pap smear or at most early precancer cells with gynecology follow-up
11. Women with both HIV and hepatitis C need a consultation with a hepatitis expert, stable liver blood tests for at least one year, and no evidence of liver scarring or cirrhosis

Source: Adapted from A. Al-Chan, J. Colon, A. Bardeguez, "Assisted reproductive technology for men and women infected with HIV," *Clin Infect Dis* 36 (2003): table 1.

before or at time of ovulation for the optimal chances of conceiving (see below).

One other option for discordant couples in which the man has HIV is to inseminate the woman with uninfected, screened donor sperm.

When Both of You Have HIV

Even when both the woman and the man have HIV, ideally they want to avoid exposure to each other's virus. One partner may have a worse or different strain of HIV than the other. To achieve pregnancy when both partners have HIV, you can follow the strategies outlined above. For example, you can inseminate washed sperm, and you can use the turkey baster method. If you decide to try for a pregnancy without help, there are two things you both can do: first, only try to achieve conception at the time of ovulation (to minimize exposure risks); and second, only try to achieve conception if you both have undetectable viral load levels.

Timing Ovulation

Ovulation refers to the moment each month when one ovary or the other releases an egg into the fallopian tube, to make its way toward the uterus. Fertilization cannot occur without the presence of a viable egg, ready for insemination and implantation. One way to predict with some accuracy when your body is ovulating is to keep a "basal temperature calendar":

- Take your temperature every morning the moment you wake up, before you arise, and before you eat or drink. Keep the thermometer convenient, next to your bed, and record each daily temperature on a graph.
- The temperature can be taken with a regular thermometer or with a special basal temperature thermometer that makes it easier to see small changes.
- Do not smoke prior to taking your temperature because this will make your temperature go up.
- When you ovulate, your temperature will increase approximately 0.5 degree F over your baseline readings.

To achieve pregnancy, you and your partner should have sexual intercourse every day starting approximately two days before your predicted ovulation and continuing until ovulation occurs. Ovulation is signaled by a rise in the basal temperature of 0.5 degree F. If you have trouble remembering to take your basal temperature, you can still estimate that ovulation will occur in midcycle. You can also purchase an over-the-counter kit to find out when ovulation occurs.

Trouble Becoming Pregnant

A couple is not considered infertile unless they have been unsuccess-fully trying to conceive a baby for over a year. Approximately 10 to 15 percent of couples in the United States are infertile. Two of the most common causes for a woman's difficulty in becoming pregnant are her age (over 35) and a history of pelvic infections. Infections like gonor-rhea and chlamydia can lead to scarring of the fallopian tubes, and this scar tissue can block each monthly egg from reaching to the uterus. Men's fertility can be decreased by soaking in a hot bath or tub, by drinking alcohol, by using drugs, and by wearing tight pants. HIV may also increase the risk for infertility. Men with low CD4 cell counts also have decreased sperm counts, poorer sperm motility (the sperm don't

Table 10.2
Initial Fertility Workup

Female
- Basal temperature diary to check for ovulation
- Follicle stimulating hormone (FSH) level test, a blood test to check if your ovaries are functioning
- Progesterone level test, a blood test drawn ideally between day 21 and 23 of a 28-day cycle to confirm that you are ovulating in the monthly cycle
- Thyroid-stimulating hormone (TSH) level test, a blood test to check the functioning of your thyroid gland

Male
- Semen/sperm analysis

Note: For a woman, a Pap smear and blood tests, including tests for rubella (measles), toxoplasmosis, syphilis, cytomegalovirus, hepatitis B, and hepatitis C may also be ordered. A hysterosalpingogram may also be considered to see whether the fallopian tubes are blocked.

move well), and more numerous abnormal sperm. It is not known whether HIV affects a woman's ability to conceive.

If you and your partner are having trouble conceiving, it is best to seek counseling from your primary care provider before you embark on a formal infertility workup or treatment. There are certain simple tests that may immediately identify the source of the problem, and if such a problem is found, you would not need an appointment with an infertility expert. For example, sperm analysis may show problems with the sperm. Or perhaps basal temperature monitoring and a test of the woman's hormone levels might reveal that she is not ovulating. Table 10.2 lists various tests your primary care provider can order to seek a reason for infertility.

Choosing among Birth Control Options

What if you don't *want* to become pregnant? Unplanned and unwanted pregnancies can be devastating experiences for women who for whatever reason do not want to conceive. Choosing the birth control method that is best for you among the many options can be a challenging task. If you know you do not want to become pregnant and you are not currently using birth control (or you are worried about how effective your birth control method is), then you will want to discuss birth control with your primary care provider. A number of considerations should be reviewed with your primary care provider before making a birth control choice:

1. How well does the method prevent pregnancy?
2. How well does the method prevent sexually transmitted diseases (STDs)?
3. Does my partner need to cooperate?
4. Do I have any medical conditions that would prevent me from using certain types of birth control?
5. Are there any side effects of the method?
6. Will the method interact with my HIV treatments?
7. Will the method affect my HIV infection?

8. Will the method affect my chances of having children in the future?

Effectiveness in Pregnancy Prevention

Many birth control methods are extremely successful at preventing pregnancy if they are used correctly. Methods shown to be more than 99 percent effective when used according to directions include hormonal methods and the intrauterine device, or IUD. Several hormonal methods have only recently become available on the market. Options include birth control pills (also known as oral contraceptives or OCPs), birth control patches (Ortho-evra), birth control shots (Lunelle shots), birth control vaginal rings (the NuvaRING), depoprovera shots (Depo shots), and Norplant implants. The newest IUD on the market, Mirena, also releases progestin or hormones. The progestin thickens the cervical mucus, suppresses ovarian function, and inhibits sperm movement, which enhances the effectiveness of this IUD.

The male and female condoms and diaphragm (which should be used with spermicides) also prevent pregnancy well, but different studies have shown that anywhere between 3 and 20 percent of women who rely on these methods alone have become pregnant. One option for women who use only condoms is to use emergency contraception (discussed in chapter 7) as a backup if the condom slips or breaks. If you want to do this, it is best to have the emergency contraception on hand, so you need to discuss this plan with your primary care provider and obtain the medications before you need them. Emergency contraception decreases the number of unintended pregnancies by about 75 percent. Spermicides give some protection against pregnancy when used alone but are most effective when used with condoms or the diaphragm.

The most effective methods for avoiding pregnancy are irreversible birth control choices. A *tubal ligation* is a surgical procedure that permanently blocks your fallopian tubes and virtually guarantees lifelong protection from pregnancy. Your male partner can undergo a very effective and less invasive surgical procedure called a *vasectomy*. This minor operation ensures that sperm cannot be released into the semen. The man will still ejaculate, but his semen will not contain sperm and therefore will not be able to fertilize an egg. Like tubal ligation, vasectomy is extremely effective but irreversible, so it would not be the right choice for someone planning to conceive children in the future.

Effectiveness in Preventing Sexually Transmitted Disease

While many hormonal birth control methods work very well to prevent pregnancy, none will protect you from catching a sexually transmitted disease like HIV or from passing an STD on to someone else. Only one method protects people from STDs: condoms. Female condoms are considered an acceptable alternative but have not been extensively evaluated for effectiveness. Spermicides give some protection against gonorrhea and chlamydia, and so does the diaphragm, but these options are not 100 percent effective against all STDs. For example, the spermicide nonoxynol-9 does not protect against HIV transmission. Therefore, condoms are *always* recommended for STD protection, even when another method of birth control is being used.

What if you *know* that you cannot get pregnant? What if you have gone through menopause or have had a hysterectomy or tubal ligation? What if you take birth control pills exactly as directed? Even if you can't get pregnant, you are still at risk for getting a sexually transmitted disease. You should still use condoms. This is true even if your partner also has HIV, because there are different strains, and one of you may transmit a more serious strain of the virus to your partner.

Of course, male condoms do require the man's cooperation. If your partner is unwilling to use male condoms, then your best protection is either to avoid having sex with him or to use female condoms with or without additional protection such as spermicides. (Female and male condoms do not need to be used with a spermicide.) *Do not* use both a male and female condom at the same time. (Additional information on condoms is found in chapter 7.)

Reversible Birth Control Methods

Oral contraceptives, or birth control pills, were the first hormonal contraceptive method that became available to women in the 1960s. The early birth control pills posed greater health risks because they contained relatively high doses of estrogen, which can increase the chances for having blood clots, strokes, and heart attacks. Today birth control pills only contain small doses of estrogen. There are still possible side effects, but the newer formulations are considered safer. Benefits, drawbacks, and possible side effects for the various hormonal methods are shown in tables 10.3 and 10.4 below.

Some women may choose not to use any hormonal method of birth control. The benefits, drawbacks, and side effects of available barrier method options are shown in table 10.5.

The IUD used to be relatively contraindicated among women with HIV because of concern regarding the potential increased frequency of pelvic infections. However, studies have shown the IUD to be safe among women with HIV, and this method is gaining acceptance. Since pelvic infections are still a possible risk factor, women who have had prior STDs may be at higher risk for this complication, and IUDs are contraindicated among women with a current, recent, or recurrent pelvic infection. Other side effects include menstrual cramping, increased bleeding during periods, and possibly making a hole in your uterus. The Mirena IUD appears to have fewer of these side effects than the older IUDs. The Mirena IUD only needs to be changed every five years, but it does require an office visit to your gynecologist.

Birth Control Methods and HIV Infection

Many hormonal birth control methods are metabolized by the same enzymes that metabolize the HIV treatment medications. For this reason, the birth control and HIV treatments may interact. HIV medicines can change the blood levels of hormonal birth control treatments, reducing their reliability. Therefore, if you are taking certain HIV treatments such as protease inhibitors, you cannot feel 100 percent secure

Table 10.3
Benefits, Drawbacks, Side Effects, Contraindications, and Dosing for Combined Estrogen and Progesterone Birth Control Methods (Includes Birth Control Pills, Ortho-evra Patch, Lunelle Shots, and NuvaRING)

General Benefits:

Decrease menstrual cramping, regulate periods, may decrease menstrual bleeding, improves acne, decreases risk for several diseases, including bone thinning (osteoporosis), ovarian cysts, ovarian cancer, uterine cancer, and pelvic infections

General Drawbacks:

Unknown effect on HIV, may increase risk of transmitting HIV to your sexual partner, interactions with HIV treatments can decrease effectiveness of method

Specific Drawbacks:

Birth control pills: Adds another daily pill

Lunelle shots: Requires office visit for shots

NuvaRING: May require practice to insert; ring may fall out

General Side Effects:

Nausea, weight gain, headaches, dizziness, breast tenderness, spotting between periods, depression; increases risk for several diseases, including blood clots, strokes, and heart attacks (especially if you smoke cigarettes)

Specific Side Effects:

Ortho-evra patch: Application site reactions (rarely)

NuvaRING: Vaginal irritation, infections, discharge

General Contraindications:

History of blood clots, uncontrolled high blood pressure, severe liver problems, breast cancer, complicated diabetes, smoker, older than 35 years

Specific Contraindications:

Ortho-evra patch: Weight more than 90 kg or 198 pounds (efficacy may be decreased)

Dosing:

Birth control pills: One pill daily

Patches: One patch a week for 3 weeks, then bleed for 1 week

Lunelle shots: One shot a month

Vaginal ring: Insert ring for 3 weeks, then bleed for 1 week

Table 10.4
Benefits, Drawbacks, Side Effects, Contraindications, and Dosing for Progesterone or Progestin Only Birth Control Methods (Includes Depo Shots, Norplant Implants)

General Benefits:
  Menstrual bleeding may stop, may decrease risks for several diseases including pelvic infections, ovarian cancer, and uterine cancer

General Drawbacks:
  Unknown effect on HIV, unknown interactions with HIV treatments and whether efficacy of method is affected

Specific Drawbacks:
  Depo: Requires office visit for shots
  Norplant: Requires procedure to insert and remove implants

Side Effects:
  Menstrual periods may become irregular or stop, weight gain, breast tenderness, depression, headaches, hair loss, increased risk for thinning bones (osteoporosis), increased risk for blood clots, possible negative effects on blood fat levels

Contraindications:
  Unexplained vaginal bleeding, breast cancer, history of blood clots, history of specific eye problems

Dosing:
  Depo shots: One shot every 3 months
  Norplant: Inserted every 5 years

in the effectiveness of birth control pills, birth control patches (Ortho-evra), birth control shots (Lunelle shots), birth control vaginal ring (NuvaRING), Depo shots, or Norplant. The only protease inhibitors that are known *not* to significantly affect the levels of birth control pills are Crixivan (indinavir) and Reyataz (atazanavir).

There is little information on whether hormonal birth control methods influence the levels of HIV treatments themselves or whether

Table 10.5

Benefits, Drawbacks, Side Effects, Contraindications, and Dosing for
Physical or Chemical Barrier Birth Control Methods
(Includes Condoms, Diaphragm, Spermicides)

Specific Benefits:

Male condom: Protects against STDs including HIV, delays premature
ejaculation

Female condom: Protects against STDs including HIV

Diaphragm: Some STD protection not including HIV

Spermicides: Some STD protection not including HIV

Specific Drawbacks:

Male condom: Needs partner cooperation, needs to be put on right before
sex

Female condom: Can be noisy during sex

Diaphragm: May require practice to insert, need to be fitted for the correct
size by gynecologist, need to use spermicide in addition to achieve best
effectiveness

Spermicides: Side effects (see below) may actually increase risk of HIV
transmission

Specific Side Effects:

Male condom: Latex allergy (but polyurethane condoms are available)

Female condom: Polyurethane allergy

Diaphragm: Latex allergy, vaginal or bladder infections, pelvic pressure,
vaginal irritation

Spermicides: Vaginal irritation, may increase risk for vaginal ulcers, vaginal
or bladder infections

Specific Contraindications:

Male condom: Latex and polyurethane allergies

Female condom: Polyurethane allergy

Diaphragm: Latex allergy

Spermicides: Allergy to any component in the spermicide

Dosing:

Male condom: With sex

Female condom: With sex, may be inserted 8 hours before sex

Diaphragm: With sex, may be inserted 6 hours before sex

Spermicides: With sex

---

they affect the HIV infection. One HIV treatment that is known to be affected by hormonal birth control methods is Agenerase (amprenavir). Agenerase levels are decreased and may be less effective against HIV when used with hormonal birth control methods, and therefore you should not use a hormonal birth control method and Agenerase together.

KEY POINTS

1. If you are sexually active, you should make an active and informed decision about whether or not to become pregnant.

2. You are most likely to get pregnant if you have sex during the middle of your menstrual cycle, between menstrual periods.

3. Both age and certain medical conditions can influence a woman's chance of becoming pregnant and can also influence the pregnancy itself.

4. If a couple wishes to conceive a baby and only one of the partners has HIV, there are ways to decrease the risk of HIV transmission to the uninfected partner.

5. When choosing a method of birth control, it is important to consider not only pregnancy prevention but also protection from sexually transmitted diseases.

6. Condoms are always recommended to prevent sexual transmission of diseases.

7. Birth control pills, birth control patches (Ortho-evra), birth control shots (Lunelle shots), deproprovera (Depo shots), birth control vaginal ring (NuvaRING), and Norplant implants are all very effective in preventing pregnancy, but each has possible side effects and their effectiveness may be decreased by HIV treatments.

8. The Mirena intrauterine device (IUD) may be an acceptable alternative birth control method for women with HIV.

11

Pregnancy

Will pregnancy affect your health if you have HIV?

What can you do to decrease the chance of transmitting HIV to your baby?

What HIV treatments can you take when you are pregnant?

Pregnancy Testing

If you are sexually active and either miss your period or have a change in your menstrual bleeding, you may be pregnant. Even if you have been using birth control, a pregnancy test is still a smart idea, because birth control methods do not always work perfectly. If you are in your early forties and you miss a period, do not assume that you are going through menopause, because women can still get pregnant at this age. The urine pregnancy tests that are available in drugstores without a prescription work very well and can detect a pregnancy very early— about two weeks after conception.

Effect of Pregnancy on HIV Infection

Women with HIV generally do well during pregnancy although their CD4 cell counts usually decrease. One reason for this may be that when a woman is pregnant, she normally has much more fluid in her body. This additional blood volume may "dilute" the number of CD4 cells. Some studies have found that changes in CD4 cell counts are the same in pregnant and nonpregnant women with HIV when they are followed over time. Other studies have found that women with HIV who become pregnant are not more likely to get sick from their HIV infection. What we can conclude from these various studies is that for many women with HIV, pregnancy does not affect the progression of disease. However, if a woman is already sick from HIV or if she has a diagnosis of AIDS, she may not be able to take all the medication she needs because of pregnancy. Some medications that she may need to treat specific AIDS infections can be dangerous to an unborn baby. Cytovene (ganciclovir) is one example. (See also "HIV Treatments during Pregnancy," later in this chapter.)

Effect of HIV on Pregnancy

Various studies designed to determine if HIV infection is related to complications in pregnancy have determined that women with HIV who are otherwise healthy do not appear to have any HIV-related pregnancy complications. On the other hand, certain complications do appear to be more common among women who are sick with their HIV infection or who also have other problems such as drug or alcohol addiction. These complications include miscarriage, poor growth of the baby in the uterus, lower birth weights, and more frequent premature deliveries. Prematurity is the most common reason babies fail to do well after they are born.

Certain infections can affect your pregnancy, and some can be transmitted to your baby. If your CD4 cell count is below 200, you should be taking antibiotics to prevent specific HIV-related conditions. Antibiotic treatment is discussed more fully in chapter 4. Infections of particular concern to pregnant women are listed in table 11.1.

Table 11.1
Infections That Affect Pregnancy

Infection	Result of Infection	Management of Infection
Genital HSV	possibly transmitted to baby at birth	treat HSV infection in mother, C-section if genital sores are present at time of delivery
Genital HPV infection or warts	possibly transmitted to baby at birth (low risk)	warts may need treatment
Syphilis	possibly transmitted to baby before birth	screen and treat mother
Hepatitis B	possibly transmitted to baby, usually at birth	screen mother and possibly treat newborns with vaccine and antibodies (immune globulin)
Hepatitis C	unclear when transmission to baby may occur; risk increased if mother has HIV	screen mother
Cytomegalovirus	possibly transmitted to baby before birth	screen mother*
Toxoplasmosis	possibly transmitted to baby before birth	screen mother and treat new infections*

Note: Hepatitis, HSV, syphilis, and HPV are discussed in chapters 5, 8, and 9.
* If a mother is newly infected with a cytomegalovirus or toxoplasmosis infection, her primary care provider will discuss treatment with her. The treatment of these infections may be different in pregnant women. (See chapter 6 for treatment of non-pregnant women.)

Transmitting HIV Infection from Mother to Baby

Fortunately, the risk of transmitting HIV infection from mother to baby has decreased dramatically in the last ten years, thanks primarily to powerful new HIV treatments. The major factors that may increase the risk of transmission are summarized in table 11.2. Controlling the

Table 11.2
Important Influences on Mother-to-Baby HIV Transmission Risk

Major Factors

Viral load level	Mothers with high viral loads are more likely to transmit HIV, but women with very low viral loads can still pass HIV to their babies.
CD4 cell count	Mothers with low CD4 cell counts are more likely to transmit HIV to their babies.
Stage of HIV	Mothers with a diagnosis of AIDS are more likely to transmit HIV to their babies.
Ruptured membranes	Mothers whose membranes rupture more than 4 hours prior to delivery are more likely to transmit HIV to their babies.
Preterm delivery	Premature babies are more likely to be infected with HIV.

Moderate Factors

Vaginal and cervical infections	Some infections may cause more HIV shedding inside the birth canal, which will increase the chances of HIV transmission from mother to baby.
Hepatitis C	Mothers who are infected with hepatitis C are more likely to transmit HIV to their babies.
Using drugs	Mothers who use drugs during pregnancy are more likely to transmit HIV to their babies.
Infection of the placenta or amniotic fluid	Mothers who have these conditions are more likely to transmit HIV to their babies.

pregnant woman's viral load is the most important factor in decreasing the chance her baby will have HIV.

It is not entirely clear whether HIV transmission is more likely to occur during pregnancy or during childbirth. It is clear, however, that certain behaviors slightly increase the risk of transmission. These include cigarette smoking and having unprotected sex with several partners during pregnancy. Vitamin A deficiency poses a transmission risk

Table 11.3
Effect of HIV Treatment on Risk of HIV Transmission from Mother to Baby

Treatment	Risk of transmission
No HIV treatment given to mother or baby	20%–25%
HIV treatment only at time of delivery with one of the options outlined in the text	9%–12%
Retrovir monotherapy for mother and baby among women with HIV viral load less than 1,000 copies	1%
Combination HIV treatment for mother and Retrovir monotherapy for baby	0–2%

Note: Studies conducted before today's powerful HIV treatments were widely available found that women taking only Retrovir had a transmission risk of 5 to 10%; these studies included women with very low CD4 counts. (Retrovir causes a 70% reduction in the rate of transmission; for women not taking any therapy, the rate of transmission is 20 to 25%.)

in countries where malnutrition is common, but it has not been identified as a risk for American women, who generally take in enough vitamin A in their diets. Routine vitamin A supplementation is not recommended during pregnancy (and will not lower the risk of HIV transmission).

Many of the risk factors for HIV transmission are under your control. The most important factors—your viral load and your general health—can be greatly improved with HIV treatments. Today's HIV treatment regimens (see chapter 6 and below) can reduce the risk of transmission to less than 2 percent when guidelines are followed and viral loads drop to undetectable levels. Table 11.3 summarizes transmission risks shown in different studies.

Vaginal versus Cesarean Delivery

A baby who has not acquired HIV during the pregnancy may become infected during delivery. Because vaginal childbirth exposes a baby to a great deal of the mother's blood, there are some situations where a cesarean section (surgical delivery) is recommended to protect the baby from HIV transmission. A C-section is recommended for any mother whose viral load is higher than 1,000. To achieve the lowest possible risk of transmission, even for a woman having a cesarean delivery, it is still critical to take HIV treatments to decrease the viral load.

A C-section is only protective when it is performed before the mother's membranes rupture—before her water breaks. Usually the C-section is scheduled at about 38 weeks to guarantee delivery before the water breaks. Women are given the drug Retrovir through a vein three to four hours before the start of the C-section.

While a C-section can reduce the risk of HIV transmission, it is a major surgery with possible complications of its own. These complications include fever, infection, anemia (low blood count), pain, and discomfort from the incision. Some of these problems, such as fever, are more likely to occur in women with HIV. Hospital stays following C-section last about five days as compared to two days after vaginal delivery.

Breastfeeding is not recommended for women with HIV infection because babies can acquire HIV infection through breast milk that contains the virus.

HIV Treatments during Pregnancy

Guidelines for beginning HIV treatments differ for pregnant and nonpregnant women. As discussed in chapter 6, nonpregnant women are generally encouraged to consider HIV treatment when their CD4 cell counts drop and/or their viral loads rise. If a nonpregnant woman is able to maintain a high CD4 count and a low viral load without treatment, she may well be encouraged to postpone treatment while continuing to have her blood work and general health closely monitored. However, a pregnant woman would receive different advice.

An extremely important study conducted in 1994 (before the widespread availability of new HIV treatments) looked at the effect of

Retrovir (also called AZT or zidovudine) on mother-to-baby HIV transmission rates and found that *Retrovir reduced the chances of transmission by 70 percent.* As a result of this study, all pregnant women are now advised to take Retrovir, even if they have low viral loads, even if they have high CD4 counts, and even if they feel generally healthy. This medicine is too beneficial to skip.

Pregnant women are encouraged to start a combination HIV treatment at lower viral loads than those who are not pregnant. (These combination regimens are described in chapter 6.) It is clear that lowering the mother's viral load through combination treatments can dramatically decrease the risk of HIV transmission to the baby. If a mother's viral load is less than 1,000 at time of delivery, the risk of transmission drops to 2 percent or less. This is why combination treatment is recommended for pregnant women with a viral load higher than 1,000. Table 11.4 outlines the treatment guidelines for pregnant and nonpregnant women.

As you can see from table 11.4, the recommended combination treatment requires that at least three different HIV treatments be given together. The exception is Retrovir, which can be given alone to pregnant women with viral loads below 1,000 and CD4 counts above 350. Some experts have raised the question of whether it is ever wise to give only one HIV treatment (called monotherapy), because there is a remote possibility that the virus may become resistant to that drug. With Retrovir this is extremely unlikely, because the virus would have to undergo several changes or mutations to outsmart this powerful drug. None of the women on Retrovir monotherapy who participated in the 1994 study developed absolute resistance to the drug, but a few women did develop minor changes in their strains of HIV that marked the first steps toward drug resistance.

For pregnant women with very low viral loads (less than 1,000) and relatively high CD4 cell counts (more than 350), the U.S. Public Health Service recommends *either* monotherapy with Retrovir *or* combination therapy (see table 11.4). Neither treatment option is necessarily superior to the other, so the final decision is left to the individual woman to make after weighing the risks and benefits of each choice with her pri-

Table 11.4
HIV Treatments for Pregnant and Nonpregnant Women
with HIV without Symptoms

	HIV treatment	
Viral load	Pregnant women	Nonpregnant women
Viral load less than 1,000 and CD4 greater than 350	Retrovir only* or combination therapy**	No HIV treatments
Viral load between 1,000 and 55,000 and CD4 greater than 200–350***	Generally combination therapy; see chapter 11	Generally no HIV treatments; see chapter 6
Viral load over 55,000 or CD4 less than 200–350	Combination therapy**	Combination therapy**

Source: U.S. Department of Health and Human Services
* Retrovir is also called AZT or zidovudine.
** Combination therapy is treatment with at least three HIV treatments.
*** Treatment should generally be offered to women with CD4 counts between 200 and 350, but this is controversial. Treatment decisions must be made on an individual basis for these women.

mary care provider. For pregnant women with viral loads over 1,000, the guidelines recommend combination therapy, or treatment with at least three HIV treatments.

Guidelines are intended to help with treatment decisions, but they cannot take into account every patient's individual health and personal circumstances. Some women with viral loads only slightly above 1,000 may reasonably opt to use Retrovir alone rather than combination therapy. All treatment plans are individualized.

Our discussion so far has assumed that women with HIV are receiving medical care, that they know their CD4 counts and viral loads, and that they have been getting prenatal care throughout their pregnancies. But what if that isn't the case? What if a woman arrives at the hospital already in labor and has no idea what her CD4 count is or even that she has HIV? Many women only learn of their HIV when they are screened during labor. There are four treatment options for pregnant women with unknown CD4 and viral load results who are already in labor:

1. Mother receives one dose of Virammune (nevirapine) at the start of labor, and her baby receives one dose of Virammune 48 hours after birth.
2. Mother receives a combination of Retrovir and Epivir (3TC or lamivudine) during labor, and her baby receives Retrovir and Epivir for one week.
3. Mother receives Retrovir only during labor through an intravenous catheter, and her baby receives Retrovir for six weeks.
4. Treatment options 1 and 3 combined.

In the United States, several studies have shown that giving the mother Retrovir during labor and then giving the baby Retrovir for six weeks starting immediately after birth will decrease the baby's chances of becoming infected with HIV. Studies done overseas have also demonstrated the benefit of giving the mother either one dose of Virammune (nevirapine) or giving her and her baby both Retrovir and Epivir (3TC or lamivudine). As already mentioned, it is difficult for HIV to become resistant to Retrovir. However, only one small change in the virus can make it resistant to Virammune or Epivir. The potential for HIV to become resistant to Virammune or Epivir is a concern for options 1, 2, and 4 listed above. In the United States, options 3 and 4 are recommended. Both seem to work equally well. All the treatments listed decrease the transmission risk to approximately 10 percent.

Assuming a woman is aware that she has HIV and that she has planned her pregnancy, when should she start HIV treatments? Generally speaking, the first twelve weeks of any pregnancy are when the baby undergoes its most intense change and development. Vital organ systems take shape early, and birth defects caused during this time can be far more serious than problems introduced later in the pregnancy after the heart and nervous system have formed. For this reason, treatment guidelines have left the decision to start HIV therapy *optional* during the first twelve weeks of pregnancy. It is not clear whether the drugs would have a significant protective effect for the baby during this period anyway. On the other hand, if a woman was already taking the medicines before she became pregnant, there may be risk associated with interrupting treatment for twelve weeks. Abruptly stopping the medications will probably cause her viral load to increase, and this increased viral activity may result in immune system damage that could heighten the risk of HIV transmission to her baby. All of these variables are still being studied and weighed against one another. Women should consult with their primary care providers in making this very personal decision.

If you become pregnant while on HIV treatments, your primary care provider and obstetrician should talk with you about any known risks for specific medications you are taking. Certain HIV treatments such as Sustiva, the liquid formulation of Agenerase, or Hydrea are known to cause problems for unborn babies. Pregnant women should also avoid the combination of Videx and Zerit, which is known to cause problems for the mother. Specific risks are discussed in more detail in chapter 6. Important considerations for anyone who becomes pregnant while taking HIV treatments are listed below.

- Women who learn of their pregnancies after the first twelve weeks of pregnancy have passed should continue taking their HIV medications.
- Women who learn of their pregnancies during the first twelve weeks can either continue taking their HIV medications or can stop all treatments until twelve weeks have passed and then start taking them again.
- Treatment regimens should include Retrovir whenever possible.
- Treatment regimens should be reviewed for the safety of both mother and baby, and any medication known to cause problems should be changed.

What if a woman starts combination HIV treatment during pregnancy, delivers her baby, and then does not meet treatment guidelines for nonpregnant women? Should she stop taking her medicines after the baby is born? Experts don't know. The woman and her primary care provider must decide. Sometimes simpler regimens that had not been recommended in pregnancy because they posed risks for the baby become good choices after delivery. One thing is clear, however: if you are taking Retrovir alone while pregnant, you should stop taking it after your baby is born.

What to Expect from Your Obstetrician Visits

Obstetricians often take on the role of primary care provider for pregnant women during their pregnancies. The current recommendation is that all pregnant women be screened for HIV because studies have shown that HIV treatment can effectively decrease the risk of transmitting the virus from the mother to the unborn child. If a woman learns she has HIV, she should have all of the blood tests described in chapter 2. The results of these tests will help guide treatment decisions during and after her pregnancy.

Other screening tests include the mother's blood type and a test for rubella (measles). Rubella can cause birth defects if the mother gets measles while pregnant. Fortunately, most women have antibodies against this disease and therefore do not need to worry about it. If you do not have antibodies against rubella, your obstetrician will explain how you should be monitored for this infection. Table 11.5 summarizes the timetable for various screening tests performed throughout pregnancy.

Certain medical conditions can increase the risk for complications during pregnancy. Examples include high blood pressure, diabetes (high blood sugar), severe anemia (low blood counts), and kidney problems. If you have any of these or other conditions that might affect your pregnancy, or if you are sick from your HIV infection, your obstetrician will probably want to start monitoring your baby sometime between 26 and 32 weeks into the pregnancy. Regular office visits and re-

Table 11.5
Timetable of Monitoring Tests during Pregnancy

Week of pregnancy	Screening test
15 to 20 weeks	Blood test to check for Down's syndrome and spina bifida
16 to 20 weeks	Ultrasound to determine the baby's age and to check for developmental defects
24 to 28 weeks	Screen for diabetes with oral glucose tolerance test*
32 to 36 weeks	Screen for vaginal and cervical infections and syphilis

Note: In addition to the screening tests listed here, women with HIV should routinely have viral load and CD4 cell count testing throughout pregnancy.

* For a glucose tolerance test, you will be asked to drink a very sugary liquid and then have your blood drawn one hour later. Women taking protease inhibitors may be at increased risk for high sugar levels. Sugar levels must be well controlled during pregnancy for the health of the unborn baby.

peated ultrasound tests will help the doctor monitor your baby's heart rate and growth and confirm that you have the right amount of amniotic fluid in your womb. You will also be monitored for contractions. At home, you can keep track of your baby's movements by counting how many you feel. You should feel at least ten movements over any two-hour period.

KEY POINTS

1. A woman on combination HIV treatment who has an undetectable viral load level is very unlikely to transmit HIV to her baby. Her chances of passing the virus to the baby are less than 2 percent.

2. Pregnancy does not appear to harm the health of women with HIV.

3. Women who are sick from their HIV infection or who have other problems such as drug addiction have a slightly higher risk for certain pregnancy complications.

4. *If a pregnant woman is sick from her HIV infection, her risk of transmitting HIV to her baby is higher than if she is well.*

5. *Even if you are pregnant, your CD4 cell count and viral load are still of central importance in deciding whether you should begin HIV treatment for your health.*

6. *Retrovir or AZT is recommended for all pregnant women with HIV because it has been proven to decrease the chance of HIV transmission from mother to baby.*

7. *A C-section may decrease the risk of HIV transmission to the baby when the mother's viral load is over 1,000.*

Resources
Pediatric AIDS Clinical Trials at www.pactg.s-3.com describes available studies for pregnant women.

12

Menstrual Periods

What causes abnormal menstrual bleeding?

How is abnormal menstrual bleeding treated?

What is the premenstrual syndrome *and how is it treated?*

Does HIV affect menstrual cycles and ovulation?

What are the symptoms of menopause and how are they treated?

Understanding Menstrual Cycles

Many of us first learned about menstrual cycles in school. If our mothers, aunts, sisters, or friends didn't fill us in, then our health teachers at least made sure we didn't experience the frightening, unexpected sight of blood without the comforting knowledge that yes, this is normal, this is healthy. The first monthly period—known as the "onset of menses" or "menarche"—is significant, for it marks the arrival of a girl's ability to become pregnant.

After she begins to menstruate, a woman generally releases one egg from either the left or right ovary each month. This process is called *ovulation*. The egg travels down the fallopian tube and into the uterus where, if it has not encountered any sperm, it will spend the next two weeks until it is shed from the body with the uterine lining that is replenished every month. If a woman has sex around the time of ovulation, then the egg may indeed meet sperm in the fallopian tube, and fertilization may take place. This will lead to pregnancy, and the uterine lining will not shed, but rather will grow in place, making a nourishing and safe place for the baby. The woman will generally not get a period that month or for eight months after that.

A normal menstrual cycle lasts from 21 to 35 days, with ovulation occurring in the middle of the cycle and the "period" of blood flow lasting two to six days at the end of the cycle. But many women do not follow this schedule. Approximately one-third of HIV-negative women have abnormal menstrual cycles. Two groups of women are most likely to experience abnormal menstrual cycles: adolescent girls who recently began to menstruate, and older women who are approaching menopause (when periods naturally stop). For both of these groups, irregular ovulation is usually the cause of the abnormal cycles. The term *anovulation* refers to a cycle in which a woman does not release an egg from her ovary at all. Anovulation is the most common cause for abnormal menstrual bleeding.

Another common cause of abnormal bleeding is uterine fibroids (tumors in the uterus). In fact, 30 percent of women with fibroids experience abnormal menstrual bleeding as their first symptom of this disorder. Other causes of abnormal cycles include certain forms of hormonal birth control, such as Depo shots or Norplant. (Birth control is discussed in chapter 10.) Hormonal medications prescribed for HIV-related symptoms, such as Megace or anabolic treatments, may also cause irregular periods. Vaginal or cervical infections, such as trichomonas or chlamydia, can cause mild vaginal bleeding, especially if there is an abnormal vaginal discharge. Table 12.1 lists additional factors that can influence menstrual cycles. But remember: if you are a sexually active woman expecting a period that doesn't arrive, you must first think of pregnancy.

If you are worried about your periods, it is important to talk with your primary care provider about your concerns. Have your periods changed? Have you missed a period? Is your blood flow heavier than

Table 12.1
Factors That Influence Menstrual Cycles

1. Anovulation (irregular periods result when no egg is released from the ovary)
2. Pregnancy or miscarriage (periods stop with pregnancy, and increased bleeding follows miscarriage)
3. Menopause (periods naturally become irregular and stop)
4. Hormone treatments* (periods may become irregular and stop)
5. Uterine fibroids (periods may become irregular or heavier)
6. Infections (may cause irregular periods and bleeding between periods)
7. Uterine or cervical cancer (may cause increased bleeding)
8. Illness (periods may become irregular or stop)
9. Profound weight loss (periods may stop)
10. Excessive exercise (periods may stop)
11. Obesity (periods may become heavier, irregular, or stop)
12. Medical disorders or medications that influence how well your blood clots (bleeding may increase)

* Including but not limited to Depo shots, Norplant, Megace, and anabolic treatments. Birth control pills generally make periods more regular.

in the past? There are reasons for such changes, and your body may be telling you something significant. For example, some women may experience abnormal bleeding as a result of an ectopic (tubal) pregnancy, which occurs when the fetus has implanted outside the uterus, generally in one of the fallopian tubes. Ectopic pregnancies cannot survive, and they become life-threatening emergencies. Do not be surprised if your health care provider advises a pregnancy test in response to your description of vaginal bleeding. Bleeding can also occur during early pregnancy because of threatened miscarriage.

The hormonal changes that accompany natural menopause can also lead to changes in menstrual bleeding. A simple blood test can check your follicle stimulating hormone (FSH) level and reveal if you are starting to go through menopause. Women who have already gone through menopause and stopped getting their periods are sometimes surprised to experience vaginal bleeding again. This is a very worrisome sign, since postmenopausal bleeding can be the first symptom of uterine cancer. Any woman who experiences postmenopausal bleeding should have a biopsy taken of her uterine lining. This is a relatively quick procedure that can be done in the gynecologist's office. The treatment for uterine cancer starts with hysterectomy, the surgical removal of the uterus, an operation that can be lifesaving.

Having irregular periods may not bother you, and if you are not having problems such as heavy or prolonged menstrual periods, you may not need to have any treatment. However, it is still important to be checked. A woman with irregular periods should find out the reason for her abnormal bleeding because abnormal vaginal bleeding can be a symptom of cervical cancer at any age, and it is a symptom of uterine cancer in women over forty.

As stated above, the most common cause of abnormal bleeding among nonpregnant, premenopausal women is anovulation. (Even healthy women with regular periods will not ovulate during 5 to 31 percent of their cycles.) When the ovaries do not release an egg each month, the hormones get out of balance. For this reason, the usual treatment for a woman who has many irregular cycles is birth control pills. The hormones in oral contraceptive pills can help regulate menstrual periods and decrease the amount of bleeding. (Chapter 10 discusses the risks and benefits of birth control pills.) If you are having heavy periods from Depo shots or from Norplant, then over-the-counter non-steroidal anti-inflammatories (NSAIDs) such as Motrin or Naprosyn may help.

If you are bothered by irregular or heavy periods, your primary care provider may suggest that you keep a menstrual calendar to record your symptoms. This calendar can help determine if your symptoms are truly abnormal and whether treatment will help. To make a menstrual calendar, simply take a regular calendar and note when your bleeding starts and stops. On the days you experience bleeding, describe it as light, medium, or heavy. Make sure to record any days when you have bleeding or spotting between your periods too.

If you have heavy abnormal bleeding because you have uterine fibroids, or if you have bleeding that does not respond to medical treatment, your primary care provider may recommend a hysterectomy. This surgery will prevent you from ever becoming pregnant. Sometimes it is possible to remove fibroids but leave the uterus in place, an operation called a *myomectomy*. Your personal symptoms and anatomy will determine whether this surgery is a reasonable option for you to consider.

What if your periods simply stop? Reasons may include pregnancy, menopause, excessive exercise, Depo shots, Norplant implants, and certain hormonal medications such as Megace. To have normal periods, a woman needs to maintain a certain weight and to stay healthy. Sometimes HIV-related complications can cause a woman to stop getting periods. But again, the most common cause for a sexually active woman to stop menstruating is pregnancy.

Premenstrual Syndrome

Nearly everyone has heard of premenstrual syndrome or "PMS." PMS refers to the mood and behavioral changes that some women experience just before the start of each period. Symptoms include a depressed or anxious mood; sudden tearfulness, anger, or sadness; and loss of interest in usual activities. Chapter 16 discusses mental health in more detail and describes how women may benefit from treatment from a mental health professional, whether with therapy, medication, or both. Useful nonmedication PMS treatments include:

- Avoiding caffeine (found in chocolate as well as coffee, tea, and soda)
- Stopping smoking
- Getting regular exercise
- Eating a healthy diet
- Getting adequate sleep
- Reducing stress

Prozac (fluoxetine) is the one prescription medication that has been shown to help with severe PMS symptoms. Alternative treatments that may help include evening primrose oil (2–4 grams) and chastberry (extract from the chast tree berry).

Menstrual Cramps and Pelvic Pain

About half of all menstruating women have cramps. The cramps can be very strong and often last two to three days. Some women also experience lower back pain, nausea, and vomiting. Because certain gynecologic conditions such as pelvic infection or ectopic pregnancy can cause pelvic pain, it is very important to see your primary care provider if your cramps are changing or getting worse. NSAIDs such as Motrin or Naprosyn will generally relieve pain that is not caused by a medical condition. Birth control pills can also help. (One study comparing women with HIV to HIV-negative women found that women with HIV were less likely to have typical premenstrual symptoms such as cramps.)

Endometriosis is a relatively common disorder that also often causes severe pelvic pain. Endometrial tissue normally lines the uterus, but a woman with endometriosis has endometrial tissue *outside* her uterus. This condition is usually diagnosed among young women 25 to 29 years of age. In addition to causing pelvic pain, endometriosis can cause infertility (difficulty becoming pregnant). Generally, endometriosis is diagnosed by laparoscopy. A laparoscope is a device that allows the gynecologist to visualize your pelvic cavity. This invention has enabled thousands of women to avoid major surgery. Laparoscopy is a comparatively minor procedure that involves making a small incision in your belly button (where the tiny scar will be hidden) and passing the narrow scope into your belly. Pelvic pain caused by endometriosis may be helped by hormonal therapy such as birth control pills. Surgical treatment of the abnormal endometrial tissue may help cure infertility caused by endometriosis.

Effect of HIV on Menstrual Cycles and Ovulation

It is unclear whether HIV infection affects menstrual cycles. There have been several studies comparing menstrual irregularities in women with and without HIV. Some studies have found no difference, but others have found that women with HIV—especially those with a CD4 cell count below 200—are more likely to have lengthy intervals between periods. These intervals might last up to six weeks. One study also showed that low CD4 cell counts and high viral loads may cause either longer or shorter menstrual cycles and irregular cycles.

There is also very little information on whether menstrual periods are affected by HIV treatments. One report from Denmark described four women who experienced increased menstrual bleeding after starting on Norvir (ritonavir). However, no other studies have found this association with Norvir. Another study that focused on the connection between HIV and menstruation found that women with HIV and regular periods do not ovulate in 29 percent of their cycles. A second study of women with HIV and both normal and abnormal periods found that 48 percent had at least one cycle in which they did not ovulate.

If a woman is trying to become pregnant, she needs to know whether or not she is ovulating. The least expensive and easiest way to determine whether you are ovulating is to keep a basal temperature calendar as described in chapter 10. You can also buy over-the-counter kits that will confirm when you ovulate.

Menopause

When women reach about forty years of age, their ovaries start producing less and less estrogen. This change in estrogen levels can cause symptoms such as hot flashes and mood changes. There are many books available to guide women through menopause—or, as some people refer to it, "the Change." While symptoms often begin in women's mid- to late forties, the average age when periods stop is 51 among HIV-negative women. Women with HIV may go through menopause earlier. One study that surveyed women with HIV found that the average age women reported for menopause was 47. Another study of twenty-four women found that two of the women reported early menopause, at ages 35 and 42, respectively.

Rarely, women go through menopause prematurely, in their thirties.

If you think this has happened to you, it is a good idea to check with your primary care provider. A blood test checking the level of a specific hormone (follicle stimulating hormone, or FSH) will confirm menopause (assuming your periods have also stopped). If your FSH level is over 40, you have gone through menopause. FSH is the hormone that stimulates your ovaries to produce estrogen. If your ovaries are not producing estrogen, the FSH level increases in your blood. Smoking may cause menopause to occur earlier.

Symptoms of Menopause

Symptoms to expect as you approach menopause include abnormal periods, hot flashes, changes in your mood and behavior, and vaginal discomfort. Many older women with HIV experience these symptoms. Another common symptom, osteoporosis, or bone thinning, is described in chapter 13.

Abnormal Menstrual Bleeding. Menstrual irregularities occur in more than half of women during the transition into menopause. Bleeding can be irregular, heavy, or prolonged. Although a change in bleeding is expected as you reach fifty years of age, it is still important to see your gynecologist whenever you notice a change in your periods because the change may *not* be due to natural menopause, but rather to a medical problem like uterine tumors or cancer. Treatments for troublesome abnormal bleeding include hormone therapies and surgery. Once you reach menopause, your periods will completely stop and vaginal bleeding should not reoccur. If it does, you need to see your primary care provider.

Hot Flashes. Hot flashes occur because of falling estrogen levels. During a hot flash, a woman experiences skin flushing, sweating, and a sensation of heat. Feelings of anxiety and rapid heart beat can also occur. Occasionally, women will experience chills after the period of flushing. The episodes usually last only one to three minutes, but they may recur five to ten times a day. Some women report having as many as thirty episodes in a day. The hot flashes may occur at night, as night sweats. Hormone therapy will successfully stop hot flashes in most women. If you are unable to take hormones, there are other medications, such as Catapres (clonidine), that may also help. If you opt not to use hormone treatment, the hot flashes should improve on their own after three to five years. Women with HIV and high CD4 counts seem to be more likely to experience hot flashes than women with low CD4 counts.

Mood and Behavioral Changes. Many women have difficulties with sleep as they approach menopause. If the sleep disturbances are related to hot flashes, hormone therapy may help. Additional treatments for sleep disturbances are described in chapter 16. Depression, anxiety, and irritability are also common symptoms during menopause. It is unclear whether these feelings result from changes in estrogen levels or from other life events that usually happen around the same time of life. For example, you may have children going through adolescence or preparing to leave home. Your own parents may be needing more support from you. These changes may be causing stress to your relationship with your partner. These sorts of significant life events naturally influence how women feel, and they often occur as women approach menopause. One study that compared women over age forty with HIV to younger women with HIV found that older women were significantly more likely to be anxious and depressed.

Vaginal Discomfort. Low levels of estrogen can affect the vagina and urethra (the tube through which you urinate). After four to five years of menopause, one-third of women who opt not to use hormone therapy experience changes in these parts of their bodies. The resulting symptoms include vaginal dryness, pain with sex, recurrent vaginal infections, pain with urination, and trouble holding urine. Hormonal therapy may help with all of these symptoms, and a woman may use topical lubricants to help relieve dryness.

Hormone Replacement Therapy

Thanks to the development of very powerful HIV treatments over the past ten years, people with HIV are now living long lives. In fact, women with HIV may have the same life spans as women without HIV and may live for nearly thirty years after menopause.

Hormone replacement therapy (HRT) may prevent or delay some of the chronic medical conditions that occur with aging. HRT may take the form of estrogen alone or of estrogen plus progesterone. You can take estrogen alone only if you have had a hysterectomy. If you still have your uterus, taking estrogen alone without progesterone increases your risk for uterine cancer.

Hormone replacement therapy can improve many of the troubling symptoms of menopause, including hot flashes, night sweats, vaginal dryness, mood swings, and trouble sleeping. It is also clear that HRT prevents bone thinning and therefore protects against broken bones. A woman's risk of colon cancer decreases if she takes HRT, and some experts suspect that her risk for Alzheimer's disease will also decrease, though the second claim requires further study.

Hormone replacement therapy also has risks, however. It has been shown to double or even triple a woman's risk of blood clots as well as to increase the risk of gallbladder disease, breast cancer (after at least five years of use), strokes, and heart attacks. Estrogen treatment without progesterone has been associated with uterine cancer as well. Less serious side effects include breast tenderness and the resumption of menstrual periods.

As explained in chapter 10, hormonal birth control interacts with HIV treatments. So does hormone replacement therapy, although there is slightly more estrogen in birth control pills than in HRT. There is no information on whether HRT affects the levels of HIV medications or if the drug interactions are significant. There is also no information on the effect of HRT on the HIV. One small study did find that HRT may improve survival among women with HIV, but this finding may have been biased because the women taking the HRT might have been seeing their primary care providers more frequently than other women and therefore keeping a closer watch on their general health.

As you can see, the simple question "Should I take hormone replacement therapy?" is actually not that simple. There are both benefits and risks with this choice. If you have bothersome symptoms from menopause and no contraindications to HRT (such as unexplained vaginal bleeding, liver disease, a personal history of blood clots, or heart disease), then it would be reasonable to consider short-term use of less than five years. The main reason women have considered long-term HRT is to prevent bone thinning. However, this benefit may not outweigh the recently identified risks associated with HRT, and health care providers are now encouraging alternative options for women who have a high risk of bone fracture. (Chapter 13 discusses bone health in greater detail.)

Hormone replacement therapy can be taken by mouth, through injections, or by a patch or a vaginal ring (Femring). If you still have your uterus, you will need to take progesterone pills in addition to receiving estrogen by an injection, patch, or vaginal ring. There are also preparations that combine the estrogen and progesterone into one pill (such as Prempro). The estrogen patches are more expensive than pills and may cause slight skin irritation. To relieve vaginal discomfort, there are moisturizing lubricants or estrogen creams to apply vaginally. These creams are sometimes recommended even for women who cannot take HRT, because the hormones applied topically are not absorbed into the bloodstream. You can discuss this option with your primary care provider.

Alternatives to Hormone Replacement Therapy

Hormone replacement therapy is not for everyone. One alternative that appeals to many women is consuming extra "phytoestrogens," which are found in a variety of plants, fruits, and vegetables such as soybeans and legumes. Phytoestrogens do not appear to have any serious side effects, and they may help with hot flashes (although a recent study found them ineffective for this purpose). They may possibly slow bone thinning. We do not know if they work as well as HRT. Phytoestrogens function in the body by binding to estrogen receptors and stimulating estrogen activity. Health food stores often carry phytoestrogens in pill form. Other alternative treatments that have been recommended for menopausal symptoms (but have not yet been proven to work) include black and blue cohosh, evening primrose oil, chastberry, licorice, and vitamin E. The FDA-approved blood-pressure medication called Catapres (clonidine) can also reduce hot flashes.

KEY POINTS

1. *Abnormal menstrual cycles occur most often in adolescents when they first start having periods and in older women who are approaching menopause.*

2. *Women with abnormal menstrual cycles are less likely to ovulate—to release an egg from one ovary each month.*

3. *Menstrual cramps and symptoms associated with premenstrual syndrome are very common and sometimes distressful. There are helpful treatments for both.*

4. *It is not clear whether HIV affects either menstrual cycles or ovulation.*

5. *Symptoms associated with menopause generally begin in a woman's mid- to late forties. These include abnormal periods, hot flashes, changes in mood and behavior, and vaginal discomfort.*

6. *Known benefits from taking hormone replacement therapy during menopause include improvement of menopausal symptoms, prevention of bone thinning, and a decreased risk of colon cancer.*

7. *Known risks from taking hormone replacement therapy during menopause include possible uterine cancer (for women who take estrogen only, without progesterone, and who have never had a hysterectomy), blood clots, gallbladder disease, breast cancer (after at least five years of use), and possibly strokes and heart attacks.*

PART FIVE

Taking Care of Yourself

Special Considerations

Staying healthy requires paying close attention to our bodies. By making careful lifestyle choices, getting regular checkups, and having special screening tests, we can make great strides in protecting our health. People with HIV can feel good and live without pain. The following chapters discuss how to take control of your future, adopt a healthy outlook, and plan for your future well-being.

13

Breast Health, Bone Health, and Heart Health

> *When should a woman start having mammograms and screening herself for breast cancer?*
>
> *How can a woman prevent osteoporosis?*
>
> *Who should have their blood fat levels checked?*
>
> *How do HIV and HIV treatments affect the risk for breast cancer, osteoporosis, or increased blood fat levels?*

Breast Health

Most women know someone who has had breast cancer. It is a very common cancer and accounts for about one-third of all cancers in women in the United States. Of all the cancers women get, only lung cancer causes more deaths in women than breast cancer. Less than 1 percent of all breast cancers occur in women under 25, but after 30 the incidence of breast cancer rises and increases with age. Women whose mother or sisters were diagnosed with breast cancer before going through menopause have a greatly increased risk of developing breast cancer.

Women with breast cancer usually have no symptoms. If they do notice anything unusual, it is typically a painless breast lump. But some women do have other symptoms: swelling, skin changes, or discharge from a nipple may all be signs of breast cancer. A persistent nipple discharge when you are not pregnant or breastfeeding is not normal, and you should mention it to your primary care provider. Many women with HIV have swollen lymph nodes, so if you feel "knots" under your arms, the swollen lymph nodes may be from the HIV infection. (Chapter 4 discusses the symptoms of HIV in more detail.) However, you should still tell your primary care provider about these knots.

Mammograms

Mammograms are X-rays that can detect slow-growing breast cancers at least two years before the lump is big enough to be felt. Having a mammogram takes about ten minutes. To obtain a clear X-ray, the mammogram technician must vigorously compress each breast against the machine. This can be uncomfortable, especially for women with breast implants, but the temporary discomfort is worth the benefit of early cancer detection.

There has been much debate about the best age to start mammogram screening. All experts agree that mammograms should be done yearly in women who are 50 years old or older. Most experts recommend mammography every one to two years for women between the ages of 40 and 50 years. If your mother or sisters were diagnosed with breast cancer when they were younger than age 40, you should begin screening with annual mammograms earlier than age 40. Mammograms are less likely to pick up breast lumps in young women because breast tissue is denser in younger women and can sometimes mask cancer. In older women, small cancers are easier to see on the mammogram images.

Breast Self-examination

Most breast cancers are first discovered by the women who have them, not by their primary care providers. It is a good idea to learn what your breasts feel like throughout a typical menstrual cycle so that you will be able to notice any unusual changes. Normally, breast tissue undergoes slight changes throughout a menstrual cycle. Your breasts can become more lumpy and tender just before your period, so experts recommend that you do your self-exam after your menstrual bleeding stops.

To do a breast self-examination, first raise one arm over your head and look in a mirror at the breast on that same side. Are there any changes that you can see? Repeat this on the other side. Next, either sit or lie down and gently press around the tissue of your entire breast with the flats of your opposite hand's fingertips. Repeat this for the other breast. You are looking for lumps. If you do this exam regularly, you will be more likely to notice changes. Also feel for any lumps or swollen lymph nodes in your armpits. If you do the self-exam in the shower, the slippery soap and water may make it easier to feel a lump.

If you or your physician has any concern about any lumps you find or your physician finds when examining you, you will probably be advised to have either a breast ultrasound study or a mammogram. The ultrasound may be a better test if you are younger than 35 years, because it is more likely to detect cancer in young, dense breast tissue.

Breast Lumps

If you have a new breast lump, it may be difficult for your health care provider to tell whether the lump is a true mass or a fluid-filled cyst. Sticking a small needle into the lump will help determine which it is. If the lump does turn out to be a mass, then a tissue sample (a biopsy) can be taken through the needle or through a minor surgical procedure.

Other conditions besides breast cancer that can cause breast lumps include a harmless condition common in women 30 to 50 years old called *fibrocystic changes*. Women with fibrocystic changes have lumpy breasts that usually become tender just before their periods. A good bra that gives adequate support can help ease the discomfort of fibrocystic changes. Some women report that cutting down on caffeine, decreasing smoking, or taking vitamin E supplements also eases the symptoms. Another noncancerous breast lump some women develop is a *fibroadenoma*. If this benign tumor gets large, your health care provider may recommend removing it, but usually fibroadenomas are simply monitored.

If you do have a breast lump that is determined to be breast cancer, you will almost certainly be referred to a surgeon. Women with HIV who get breast cancer tend to have unusual forms of breast cancer and a rapid progression of the disease. In addition to surgery, hormonal therapy, chemotherapy, and radiation therapy may be recommended for the most aggressive possible treatment.

Bone Health

Osteoporosis

When we were children, our bones were busy gaining length, thickness, and strength. We gained weight and our bones grew stronger. As adults, if we pursue sports like weight lifting or if our jobs require weight-bearing exercise, our bones benefit from this extra challenge. Normally, however, women's bones begin to thin as we age through our thirties. This process accelerates after menopause, and women who do not take hormone replacement therapy can lose up to 5 percent of their bone tissue every year. Thin bones are more likely to break or fracture. A broken back bone or broken hip can be a very serious injury, especially in old age. Therefore, *osteoporosis*—or severe bone thinning—is a condition of great concern for all women.

Thin women have a higher risk for fractures than heavy women, and smokers have a higher risk than nonsmokers. Caucasian women have a higher risk for fractures than African-American women, and anyone with a personal or family history of hip fractures is also at higher risk. People with HIV, especially those who have taken HIV treatments and who have glucose or sugar problems (such as a tendency toward diabetes), have appeared to be at higher risk for osteoporosis than people without HIV. Protease inhibitors were the specific group of HIV treatments especially associated with this problem. However, a recent study found protease inhibitor use for at least one year to be protective against bone loss. So it is not clear if, why, or how bones are affected by either the virus or HIV treatment.

Once lost, bone cannot be replaced. Therefore, early detection is important. How do you know if you have osteoporosis? The best screening test to determine how strong your bones are is called a *DEXA scan*, which stands for dual energy X-ray absorptiometry scan. DEXA scans are superior to regular X-rays. A regular hip X-ray, for example, will only reveal very severe bone thinning after a person has already lost more than 30 percent of her bone mass. The National Osteoporosis Foundation recommends DEXA scans for women 65 years and older who are considering treatment for osteoporosis as well as for younger women who have gone through menopause, have at least one risk factor, and are considering treatment.

Quantitative ultrasound methods are being used more and more frequently to assess bone thinning. Taking a measurement on a person's heel bone can identify who may already have osteoporosis.

Prevention and Treatment of Osteoporosis

In addition to weight-bearing exercise, there are other things women can do to build up their bones against future loss. Adequate calcium intake is important. Vitamin D helps the body absorb calcium, so the two are generally taken together. (Milk is fortified with vitamin D and our bodies naturally make vitamin D when our skin is exposed to sunlight.) Women who are not on hormone replacement therapy (HRT) should take 1,500 mg calcium-plus-vitamin D supplements every day. Women on HRT can reduce this dose to 1,200 mg calcium-plus-vitamin D supplements each day. Ideally the pills should be taken at meals, with a full glass of water. It is best to take only 600 mg at a time, for example 600 mg twice daily or 500 mg three times daily.

Hormone treatments can help prevent osteoporosis (these treatments are explained in chapter 12). However, taking HRT has risks that need to be weighed against the benefits. Other, nonhormonal, medical treatments are also available for osteoporosis. A class of medicines called *bisphosphonates* is effective for both preventing and treating osteoporosis. Fosamax (also known as alendronate) is a bisphosphonate. These drugs have been shown to decrease the risk for bone fractures by 50 percent. Selective estrogen receptor modulators (such as Evista, also called raloxifene) are medications that make the spine and hip bones stronger. Women who take Evista have a 30 percent lower risk for breaking bones in their back. These medications will not help other symptoms from menopause such as hot flashes, but they are effective for prevention and treatment of osteoporosis. They pose no increased risk for uterine or breast cancer, but Estiva does raise the risk for blood clots.

Osteonecrosis

People with HIV have a higher chance of being diagnosed with *osteonecrosis* than people without HIV. Osteonecrosis refers to bone death, and is not related to osteoporosis. Having one of these conditions does not increase the risk for the other. Usually osteonecrosis occurs in the hip. The increased incidence of osteonecrosis in people with HIV may be due to the effect of HIV treatments on blood fat levels, and HIV treatments may increase certain blood fat levels. A high triglyceride level, for example, is a known risk factor for osteonecrosis. Steroids, frequently given for certain HIV-related complications, can also increase the risk. Thus it is not clear whether the increased risk of osteonecrosis is due to HIV treatments or to the virus itself. Pain medications are usually prescribed for any discomfort related to the condition, and joint replacement surgery may be necessary at some point. If you have persistent unexplained joint pain, your provider may wish to order an X-ray to determine whether you have osteonecrosis.

Heart Health

Like breast cancer and osteoporosis, heart disease is a serious problem for thousands of women. It is a top cause of death in the United States for both women and men. Fortunately, a great deal of research has helped us identify risk factors for heart disease as well as how to prevent and treat its many forms. Listed below are the characteristics known to place a person at risk for having a heart attack.

1. Diabetes
2. Certain blood vessel diseases
3. Age (men over 45 years, women over 55 years)
4. Family history of heart disease (brother or father with heart disease before age 55, or mother or sister with heart disease before age 65)
5. Current cigarette smoker
6. High blood pressure
7. High LDL blood fat levels

People with diabetes or certain blood vessel diseases (1 and 2) are at highest risk. Over a period of ten years, their cumulative risk for having a heart attack is 20 percent.

Notice that the last factor listed is "high LDL blood fat levels." LDLs—or low-density lipoproteins—are more commonly known as "bad cholesterol." All adults should have their blood fat levels checked at some point, but people taking certain HIV treatments (protease inhibitors) need to be especially vigilant about screening because protease inhibitors can cause unwanted changes in blood fat levels.

The usual screening test for blood fat is the total cholesterol level. If your total cholesterol level is high, you should have additional blood tests done to check specific fat levels. In addition to the total cholesterol, the other blood fat levels that should be checked are triglycerides (which you want at a low level), low-density lipoprotein (LDL) cholesterol (which you also want at a low level), and high-density lipoprotein (HDL) cholesterol or "good cholesterol" (which you want at a high level). Unfortunately, HIV treatments often cause all these levels to head in the wrong direction: HDLs drop, while LDLs and triglycerides rise. So blood fat levels should be regularly monitored when you take these therapies.

Even if you are not taking HIV treatments, it is a good idea to check your cholesterol levels as you age. The U.S. Preventive Services Task Force recommends that all men at least 35 years old and women at least 45 years old be screened. If you have any of the other risk factors for heart disease listed above, you should consider having cholesterol screening at an even earlier age. For accuracy, the screening blood test requires you to fast for twelve hours before having your blood drawn, so people often choose to schedule this test early in the morning and bring breakfast with them so they don't have to be hungry for long. If your levels are elevated, you may require medications to lower the triglycerides, total cholesterol, and LDL cholesterol.

Who Needs Treatment for Abnormal Blood Fat Levels?

For some people, changes in lifestyle can normalize blood fat levels without the need for medication. If your levels are only slightly elevated and you do not have other risk factors for heart disease, then simply eating a low-fat diet, exercising regularly, losing weight if indicated, and quitting smoking may do the trick. These recommendations are heart-protective and wise for all people, regardless of their blood fat levels.

For some people, however, medical treatment is also advised. Table 13.1 describes the LDL levels that health care providers use as thresholds when deciding whether to start medications. The table is a bit complicated because not everyone requires medication at the same LDL level. Someone with diabetes, for example, should begin medication at an LDL level of 130 or above, with a goal of reducing the LDL level to 100. However, a person without diabetes who has fewer than two of the risk factors listed in this chapter would not start medications unless her LDL level reached 190, and then her goal would be to reduce the level to 160. High triglycerides alone may be reason to start medication in some people even if the LDL level is okay.

The medications most frequently used to treat high blood fat levels are called *statins*. Unfortunately, certain HIV treatments (protease inhibitors) may interact with statin drugs, increasing the blood levels of the statins. Therefore, it is generally best to use only low doses of

Table 13.1
Medication Thresholds for Abnormal Blood Fat Levels

Health status	LDL level at which medication is recommended	Goal LDL
For people without heart disease, diabetes, or specific blood vessel diseases		
and fewer than two risk factors	190	160
and two or more risk factors	130–160*	130
For people with any of the following conditions: heart disease, diabetes, specific blood vessel diseases, multiple risk factors creating overall high risk		
	over 130**	100

* People at higher risk should have medication started at LDL levels of 130.
** Some experts even advise starting medication at LDL levels between 100 and 129 for people with heart disease, diabetes, specific blood vessel diseases, or multiple other risk factors.

statins if you are taking protease inhibitors. The two statins least likely to interact with protease inhibitors are the drugs Pravachol (pravastatin) and Lipitor (atorvastatin). The main side effect of statins is muscle soreness. If you develop sore muscles, mention this problem to your health care provider. The medication most commonly prescribed to treat elevated triglyceride levels is called Lopid (gemfibrozil). Fortunately, protease inhibitors do not appear to significantly affect Lopid levels.

KEY POINTS

1. Starting at age 40, women should have mammograms to screen for breast cancer. If a woman's mother or sister was diagnosed with breast cancer before the age of 40, she should begin mammogram screening earlier.

2. You should do a breast self-examination every month and visit your provider if you feel a lump or an area of change.

3. *Your bones will start thinning after you reach 30 years of age, and the rate of thinning will increase after you go through menopause. Calcium supplements and weight-bearing exercise will help slow the bone thinning.*

4. *HIV infection appears to increase the risk of bone thinning (osteoporosis) and of bones dying (osteonecrosis).*

5. *There are several treatments to prevent and treat bone thinning, including hormone replacement therapy (discussed in chapter 12).*

6. *Certain HIV treatments may affect your blood fat levels. Specific elevated blood fat levels can increase your risk for a heart attack.*

7. *You should have your blood fat levels checked if you are on HIV treatments. Treatments for elevated blood fat levels include diet and exercise as well as medications.*

14

Alcohol Dependence, Drug Addiction, and Treatment

How can you tell if you are addicted to drugs or alcohol?

If you are addicted to drugs or alcohol, what can you do to recover?

Will you get withdrawal symptoms if you stop using drugs or alcohol?

How does a pregnant woman's drug or alcohol use affect her unborn baby?

How does methadone interact with HIV treatments?

Drug and Alcohol Dependence and Addiction

Anyone can become addicted to alcohol or drugs, legal or illegal. It does not matter how much money you have, what you do for a living, or what you look like. If you have a problem with drugs or alcohol, you are not alone. An estimated 7.5 million women in the United States are addicted to alcohol, and many women are addicted to drugs. This enormous number still does not take into account everyone affected by these addictions. The families, co-workers, and friends of people addicted to drugs or alcohol also suffer. The good news is that help is available to anyone who wants to find freedom from addiction.

As with so many challenges in life, the first step toward recovery is recognizing the problem. Sometimes it helps to ask yourself the blunt question: Am I an addict? Am I an alcoholic? Again, it doesn't matter if you're a movie star, a teacher, a diplomat, or a homemaker, the question is the same. The importance of this harsh and direct question is that it is often the most powerful motivator for recovery. When someone can admit to herself that she has a serious problem with drugs or alcohol, she is ready to learn more about addiction and about how to escape it.

Some people wonder if it is possible to become addicted to drugs that are prescribed to them by their primary care providers. Here it is critical to understand the difference between "dependence" and "addiction." If you are chronically prescribed certain strong pain medications, your body may indeed become physically dependent on them. However, even if you are physically dependent on these medications, you are not an addict unless you begin to use the drugs more frequently or at higher doses than your doctor instructs and the drugs start to become a focal point of your life.

If you spend the majority of your time thinking about and using the pain medication, recovering from the effects, and trying to obtain more, and if you find that your work and social life are affected by your use of the pain medication, then yes, you may be addicted to prescription drugs. The following checklist will help you determine if you have a drug or alcohol problem. Check off those that apply to you.

❑ Over time, have you noticed that you need more drugs or alcohol to get high? For example, does drinking a six-pack give you less of a buzz than it did a year ago?

❑ Do you get withdrawal symptoms (described below) when coming off the drug or if you don't get a drink?

❑ Do you feel you are using drugs or alcohol more than you should?

❏ Have you been unsuccessful when you try to cut down or stop your drinking or drug use?

❏ Is your work or social life affected by your drinking or drug use?

❏ Do friends or family members complain about your drinking or drug use?

❏ Do you continue to drink or use drugs even though you know your behavior is causing problems?

If you checked three or more boxes, you may have a problem, and you should seek help from your primary care provider. By answering honestly and admitting that you may have a drug or alcohol problem, you have already taken the first step toward solving it.

If you are worried about taking any pain medication, keep in mind that only very rarely does a person with no history of drug or alcohol abuse become addicted to prescription pain medication. You should not let fear of addiction stop you from seeking pain relief if your doctor recommends pain medications.

Commonly Used and Abused Substances

People can develop problematic habits with all sorts of drugs, but the specific substances described below are the most common substances for abuse and addiction among women with HIV.

Heroin and Other Narcotics

Heroin is an example of an *opioid* drug, that is, a drug made from opium poppies (a flower), and is part of a class of drugs called *narcotics*, which have the potential for abuse. Examples of opioid prescription drugs are Tylenol 3, Demerol, Dilaudid, Percocet, Percodan, Vicoden, Lortab, Oxycontin, Tylox, Talacen, Talwin, and MS Contin.

Many people like using heroin or other opioids for the high they produce. Some people say that when they use these drugs, their everyday problems seem to melt away, leaving them happy, relaxed, and even euphoric. When heroin is injected, the euphoria (or extreme happiness) begins nearly immediately, lasts for about an hour, and is followed by one to four hours of sleepiness before withdrawal symptoms start. These symptoms include:

- Anxiety, nervousness, restlessness, irritability, agitation
- Nausea or vomiting
- Muscle aches
- Runny nose, teary eyes
- Dilated pupils
- Sweating
- Diarrhea
- Yawning
- Fever
- Shivering

These withdrawal symptoms are very uncomfortable. To avoid them, people turn once again to the drug. This is how the cycle of addiction begins.

When managed by a prescribing physician, opioids can be safely used to vastly improve the quality of life for people with chronic pain. While these narcotics do not cure the cause of the pain, they allow people not to care about the pain. All prescription narcotics have abuse potential, but it is extremely rare for someone to become addicted to these medications if they are taken appropriately under a doctor's supervision. For a person with a personal history of overusing drugs or alcohol, however, the risk of addiction to prescription opioids is higher. If this applies to you, you should discuss potential physical dependency with your primary care provider before taking any of these medications.

Cocaine/Crack

Cocaine is an extremely addictive drug. The euphoric high that comes from smoking crack cocaine occurs within a few seconds, leaving the user feeling energized and powerful. The drug can be snorted, injected, or smoked. Once the high has worn off, the user has intense cravings for more of the drug. These cravings often cause users to become aggressive and agitated. They often have impaired judgment and an increased willingness to take risks—a bad combination. Cocaine is very dangerous because of the rapid high and the feelings of invincibility and power it produces. In fact, users "rev up" their bodies so much with the drug that they sometimes have heart attacks, even at very young ages. Cocaine is not prescribed for any medical purpose.

Marijuana

Marijuana is widely used in the United States and may have medical benefits for some people with HIV and other diseases by helping to reduce nausea and promote appetite. Marinol (dronabinol) is the prescription derivative of marijuana that many doctors prescribe to control their patients' nausea or weight loss. Some people with these symptoms say that smoking marijuana works better for them than taking Marinol, because they have better control over the dose. People generally use marijuana to relax and to elevate their mood, but the drug can also cause drowsiness and a feeling of apathy, or not caring about anything.

Alcohol

Alcohol is a widely advertised and cheerfully packaged legal drug that is just as dangerous and addictive as many illegal drugs. People often turn to alcohol to help them relax and feel less inhibited. Alcohol can kill liver and brain cells, and people who chronically drink large amounts of alcohol may develop cirrhosis or liver failure. (Cirrhosis refers to irreversible scarring of the liver.)

Protecting the liver from inflammation is extremely important for anyone taking HIV treatments. Liver function tests are monitored regularly. Although there is no known direct interaction between alcohol and these medications, both can affect the liver. If the liver becomes too inflamed, HIV treatments may need to be stopped, possibly allowing increased viral load and subsequent immune system damage to develop. These are high prices to pay for alcohol dependence, and therefore alcoholism is a very important problem to address with your primary care provider.

If you have developed a physical dependence to alcohol and stop drinking, you may experience the following withdrawal symptoms:

- Nervousness
- Rapid heart beat
- Shaky hands
- Trouble sleeping
- Nausea or vomiting
- Sweating
- Possibly hearing or seeing things that aren't there
- Possibly seizures

Drugs, Alcohol, and Pregnancy

If you are pregnant, drugs and alcohol can have serious unwanted effects on your unborn baby, ranging from poor growth to severe mental retardation. Table 14.1 describes some of the problems substance abuse can cause in pregnancy.

Treatment for Drug or Alcohol Dependency

People addicted to drugs or alcohol lose control over their lives. Their physical health suffers, and their mental health suffers. But help is available. The first and biggest step toward treatment and recovery is recognizing that you have a problem. The providers that care for you realize how difficult it is to fight addiction and will help you however they can. Many clinics who care for people with HIV have addiction treatment centers and support groups. Some residential treatment centers and outpatient day programs accept women and their young children.

Table 14.1
How Drugs and Alcohol May Affect an Unborn Baby

Heroin or Other Opioid/Narcotic Drugs
   The baby will become physically dependent on the drug while in the
      womb and will suffer withdrawal symptoms after birth.

Cocaine/Crack
   The baby has a higher chance of being born too early.
   The baby will grow more slowly.
   The baby's head will not grow as well as it normally would.
   The baby's brain may not develop as it normally would.*

Alcohol
   Alcohol can cause fetal alcohol syndrome (FAS).**

* Part of the unborn baby's brain can even die, because cocaine can slow or temporarily stop blood flow in the baby's brain.
** Babies with fetal alcohol syndrome have slower growth, smaller heads, and heart problems. Some babies with FAS have severe mental retardation.

Addiction is a lifelong problem. Staying clean for a limited time does not mean that you are "cured." If you are addicted to drugs or alcohol, you will constantly need to fight your addiction. Be proud of yourself for seeking needed help, and be proud of any time that you are able to turn away from drugs or alcohol.

Many people addicted to drugs or alcohol also suffer from depression or anxiety. There is no shame in this. If your mental health problem is treated at the same time as your addiction, addiction relapse is less likely, and you will regain better control of your life more quickly. Keeping this in mind, your mental health or primary care provider will help you choose the drug or alcohol treatment that best answers your needs. Table 14.2 lists various available treatment options. Many people rely on a combination of these.

Table 14.2
Treatment Options for Drugs or Alcohol Dependency

Psychological Support
- Individual therapy
- Group counseling
- Family therapy

Medications for Specific Substance Dependencies
- Dolophin (methadone), for heroin/narcotics
- LAAM (1-alpha-acetyl-methadol), for heroin/narcotics
- Buprenex (buprenorphine), for heroin/narcotics
- Narcan (naloxone), for heroin/narcotics
- Antabuse (disulfiram), for alcohol
- Zyban (bupropion), for cigarettes

Self-help Programs*
- Narcotics Anonymous
- Cocaine Anonymous
- Alcoholics Anonymous
- Women in Sobriety

Inpatient and Outpatient Rehabilitation Programs**

* Self-help programs provide psychological support.
** Rehabilitation programs provide psychological support and sometimes medications as well.

Treatment Programs for People Addicted to Heroin or Other Narcotics

All people who chronically use opioids or other narcotics will become physically dependent on these drugs or medications. If a physically dependent person suddenly stops taking the particular substance her body has come to expect, she will experience some of the withdrawal symptoms listed above. That is why it is so difficult for heroin users to simply turn their backs on the drug. It is a very rare person who can quit using heroin without help.

To help heroin users recover from their addiction, the drug Dolophine (methadone) is often prescribed to prevent withdrawal symptoms. This is a carefully controlled medication. Once a person starts taking Dolophine (methadone), her dose can be slowly decreased over time until she either takes a stable low dose or stops taking methadone altogether. Some people with severe heroin habits continue to take this medication for the rest of their lives to maintain control over their addiction.

Methadone works because it frees people from the highs and lows of the heroin cycle and gradually eliminates the drug craving. It has been shown to change the lives of people addicted to heroin. Methadone maintenance treatment programs determine the particular dose each participant needs to suppress withdrawal symptoms. In addition to providing the medication, these treatment programs offer individual or group counseling. The long-term goal of methadone-maintenance programs is to avoid having participants relapse back into heroin or other narcotic abuse.

For people with HIV, it is important to realize that Dolophine (methadone) can interact with HIV treatments. Anyone taking HIV treatments who enrolls in a methadone-maintenance program needs to let the program know about her HIV treatment and likewise needs to make sure her primary care provider knows about the methadone. Adding medications or changing the dose of any medication may affect the required dose of other medications. Table 14.3 lists known interactions between commonly used HIV treatments and Dolophine (methadone).

Methadone is not the only medication available to help prevent the withdrawal symptoms that follow opioid use. LAAM (*l*-alpha-acetylmethadol) is an opiate similar to methadone that can block the effects of heroin for up to three days. Unlike methadone, which is taken every day, LAAM only needs to be taken three times each week. Another medication called Buprenex (buprenorphine) has the same effect as methadone but is given as a shot. Narcan (naloxone), a medication that stops the pleasurable effects of heroin or other narcotics, is used in emergency rooms to stop people taking opiates and in that way save lives threatened by heroin overdose.

Table 14.3
Interactions between Methadone and Common HIV Treatments

Rifadin (rifampin)	Rifadin decreases methadone levels
Mycobutin (rifabutin)	Mycobutin decreases methadone levels
Retrovir (zidovudine)	Methadone increases Retrovir levels
Norvir (ritonavir)	Norvir decreases methadone levels by 37%
Viracept (nelfinavir)	Viracept may decrease methadone levels
Kaletra (lopinavir)	Kaletra may decrease methadone levels by 53%
Virammune (nevirapine)	Virammune decreases methadone levels
Sustiva (efavirenz)	Sustiva decreases methadone levels

Treatment Programs for People Addicted to Cocaine

Generally speaking, people who use cocaine really like it. They like it so much that their old friends fall by the wayside, their family members often stop supporting them, they stop doing things they once loved to do, and their entire lives start to revolve around obtaining and using cocaine. It is very difficult for people to give up cocaine. When someone decides to stop using cocaine, the best first step may be a short stay in the hospital to help with the detoxification process—especially if the person is high at the time. Hospitalization also removes the person from whatever environment tempted her to keep using drugs. Many people find a hospital stay extremely helpful; other people wish to avoid hospitalization. For all of these people, counseling and support are necessary steps to recovery.

Counseling usually helps a person think about all aspects of her life and identify the people, places, and things associated with her cocaine habit. Sometimes women realize that recovery will require them to move out of their own homes, where the drug use or drug dealing is known to take place. Counselors can help people identify "true friends" and enjoyable activities, and can help heal families. Certain medications like the beta-blocker Inderal (propranolol) have been shown to help some people stay in treatment longer and use less cocaine in the future. Recovery from drug addiction may be a difficult hike, but it will never be regretted.

Treatment Programs for People Addicted to Alcohol

Alcoholism can become life-threatening even for those who never drink and drive. As described above, the withdrawal symptoms that follow when an alcoholic person abruptly stops drinking can be quite serious. For this reason, treatment for alcoholism should involve a "detox" program. Detoxification units monitor withdrawal symptoms and are ready with medical treatment if it is needed. The usual treatment for alcohol withdrawal symptoms is a benzodiazepine such as Valium, which can be given in lower and lower doses over time. (For more information on benzodiazepines, see chapter 16.)

Once a person has completed detoxification and has no more alcohol in her bloodstream, she can be referred to an inpatient or outpatient rehabilitation program. Rehabilitation programs often incorporate the use of a medication called Antabuse (disulfiram), which works by making a person feel very nauseated if she drinks alcohol while taking the drug. However, Antabuse only works if it is taken daily, and not all people have the necessary motivation to follow through, take the pills every day, and allow the medicine to do its job effectively.

Treatment Goals

Addiction can be managed, but it never goes away. It is a problem that requires lifelong vigilant monitoring and control. The goal of all drug and alcohol treatment programs is to help people stay drug- and alcohol-free for as long as possible while always remembering the risk of relapse. Not everyone shares the same triggers for relapse.

Each person who has experienced drug or alcohol addiction needs to recognize her own risk factors and identify her own temptations. These may include certain places or certain friends. It may be hard to stay away, but often that will be the only solution. It is critical to find a primary care provider you feel comfortable talking with—a non-judgmental person who will offer meaningful treatment options.

Everyone with a drug or alcohol problem should seek professional help. The gains can be tremendous.

KEY POINTS

1. *Treatment options for people addicted to drugs or alcohol include self-help programs, rehabilitation programs, psychological support, and medication.*

2. *For people addicted to heroin or alcohol, severe and dangerous withdrawal symptoms can result from abruptly stopping use of these substances.*

3. *Drugs and alcohol can affect a pregnant woman's unborn baby.*

4. *Methadone interacts with several HIV treatments. Anyone taking both methadone and HIV treatments should have her medication levels monitored carefully.*

Resources

National Clearinghouse for Alcohol and Drug Information (NCADI) at www.health.org/pubs/hivaids.htm or www.health.org/pubs/catalog/intr.htm or call 1-800-729-6686.

15

Intimate Partner Violence and Abuse

> *How can you tell if you are being abused?*
>
> *What actions can you take if you are being abused?*

Intimate partner violence, also known as domestic violence, is more common than most people realize. In fact, it is an extremely serious problem of epidemic proportions. For example, when a large group of women were polled (most of whom had HIV), two out of every three respondents said they had personally experienced domestic violence. Thirty percent of all female murder victims were killed by a current or former intimate partner, compared to the 2 percent of male murder victims who were killed by an intimate partner. No group of people is immune to intimate partner violence. It affects people of different age groups, religions, races, ethnicities, socioeconomic levels, educational backgrounds, and sexual orientations.

But what exactly *is* intimate partner abuse? Is it when a man hits his girlfriend? What if he hits her but leaves no marks? What if he just shouts and curses at her? What if he holds her in his arms and tells her that she is no good and will never amount to anything? Or he threatens to stop providing financial support for their children if she leaves? Or he takes her paycheck? The answer may surprise some readers: *every one of these scenarios is an example of intimate partner abuse.*

Intimate partner abuse occurs when a current or former romantic partner, either male or female, mistreats the other partner. The abuser is seeking control of the partner. Abuse is about control, and control can take many forms. Most people see that hitting or raping another person is abusive. However, more subtle kinds of abuse, such as emotional abuse, can be just as damaging.

Many people who are being verbally or emotionally abused do not even recognize the abuse. They have grown accustomed to this controlling treatment from another person and may even consider it normal. The intimate violence checklist in table 15.1 can help you find out if you are in an abusive relationship. If you answer "yes" to any of the items in the checklist, you may be a victim of intimate partner violence.

While physical abuse occasionally happens "out of the blue," it usually begins with "put downs," threats, and cursing and only later esca-

Table 15.1

Recognizing Abuse

Does your partner

❑ insult you in front of your friends or family?

❑ put down your accomplishments or goals?

❑ make you feel like you are unable to make decisions?

❑ use intimidation or threats to gain compliance (including threatening you, your family, or your pets or threatening to hurt himself or herself)?

❑ tell you that you are nothing without him or her?

❑ shove you, slap you, or hit you?

❑ call you several times a night or show up to make sure you are where you said you would be?

❑ use drugs or alcohol as an excuse for saying hurtful things or abusing you?

❑ blame you for the abuse?

❑ tell you that jealousy is a sign of love?

Table 15.1 (*continued*)

❏ pressure you sexually for things you aren't ready for?

❏ make you feel like there is "no way out" of the relationship?

❏ control who you see, what you do, or where you go?

❏ try to keep you from leaving after a fight or leave you somewhere after a fight to "teach you a lesson"?

❏ try to control your money?

❏ destroy your personal belongings?

❏ make all the decisions?

❏ tell you to dress a certain way?

Do you

❏ sometimes feel scared of how your partner will act?

❏ constantly make excuses to other people for your partner's behavior?

❏ believe that you can help your partner change if only you changed something about yourself?

❏ try not to do anything that would cause conflict or make your partner angry?

❏ feel as if no matter what you do, your partner is never happy with you?

❏ always do what your partner wants you to do instead of what you want to do?

❏ stay with your partner because you are afraid of what your partner would do if you broke up?

❏ show up late for work because you had a fight with your partner?

❏ make excuses for your partner's behavior?

❏ have to hide your bruises from your friends, co-workers, and family?

Source: Adapted from *Reaching & Teaching Teens to Stop Violence,* Nebraska Domestic Violence Sexual Assault Coalition, Lincoln, NE, April 1996, and from the Corporate Alliance to End Partner Violence, Bloomington, IL, http://www.caepv.org.

lates into physical violence. Usually after an episode of physical violence, a period of time will pass when the abusing partner says that he or she is sorry and appears to be genuinely remorseful. The abusing partner may be very sweet during this time, doing chores that he or she does not usually do, taking the abused partner out to dinner, and so on. This phase of the "cycle of violence" is often called the "honeymoon period" because it can seduce the abused partner into thinking that the trouble has passed.

Who May Be an Abuser?

Don't be fooled by a pleasant appearance. Anyone, no matter how good-looking, can be an abuser. It is important to learn to recognize the warning signs that you may be involved with an abuser. Many of these warning signals have to do with your partner's attitude. For example, abusive men tend to lack respect for women. They often think of women more as objects to be used for their own ends than as people. Also, abusers often make excuses for their behavior by blaming it on other things. An abusive partner may say something like, "I had a bad day at work"—as if a bad day at work somehow justifies mistreating another person. Abusive men often drink too much alcohol, have poor self-esteem, and have problems resolving conflicts. They are jealous and possessive. As children, many abusive men were cruel to animals. Many abusive men were victims of abuse themselves.

Why Do Women Stay with Abusers?

This question sounds simple, but the answers to it are complicated. Because just asking the question shows no understanding of what it means to be caught in an abusive relationship, many abused women find the question annoying or overwhelming. Where to begin? Women do not intentionally "sign up" for abuse, and if abuse were easy to recognize, understand, and escape, domestic violence would be a rare thing. The thousands of women who remain entangled with abusive men feel stuck for many reasons. They may not even fully understand why they don't leave.

For starters, abuse often begins on an emotional level, with the abuser chipping away at his partner's self-esteem. A woman who for years has been told that she is worthless or stupid or that she would never be able to make it on her own may ultimately start to doubt herself. Perhaps as a child she was given these hurtful messages by an abusive parent, and now her partner is telling her the same things. It makes sense that she would lack self-confidence. To complicate the situation further, this same abusive partner might at other times say very loving things to her. After an episode of verbal or physical abuse, he might apologize, declare his love, and say that he will never again do anything to hurt her. These are words she wants to hear and very much wants to believe. He may be persuasive, and his words may seem heartfelt and full of remorse. She may, as a result, believe him. She is hoping and praying that things will get better.

But will things really improve? Not if the abuser refuses to recognize that he has a problem and that he needs professional help. Too often women blame themselves for the domestic violence. They may resolve to "be better" and to somehow behave in a way that is less likely to trigger the abuse. Sadly, this plan never works, because the abuse comes from inside the abuser, not from the victim. In addition, women often wonder if they are being "too sensitive" or if they are "overreacting." It is important to recognize that these feelings are constantly encouraged by the abuser, who minimizes the violence and throws the victim's judgment into question. Keeping a diary of all instances that you perceive as abuse can help you see the abuse more clearly and stop doubting yourself.

If your partner recognizes that he or she is an abuser and is motivated to change, your relationship may have a chance. Unfortunately, many partners persist in denying that they are abusive. Others may admit the abuse but refuse to get help or change their behavior. Most professionals who work with victims of intimate partner abuse do not recommend couples therapy at first. Joint counseling will not help much if the abusive partner is unwilling to try to change. The abusive partner, not the relationship, is the problem. Therefore, experts suggest that the abuser first seek treatment alone and then, upon successful completion of treatment, consider couple's therapy. Even if your partner refuses to seek treatment, you are still likely to benefit from your own individual psychotherapy or from crisis counseling. The National Domestic Violence Hotline at 800-799-SAFE (7233) can direct you to professionals near you who specialize in treating victims of intimate partner abuse.

Even if they are emotionally ready, women often are unable to leave their partner because of practical reasons. Many abused women have little money and few social resources, and they don't know where to go. Many also have children. Women with children often worry that they won't be able to meet their children's needs if they choose to relocate without adequate resources. Some also feel it is wrong to separate the children from their father. However, it is always better for children to be in a single-parent household without abuse than in a dual-parent household where abuse is occurring. Children are traumatized by living in violent households, whether or not the violence is directly targeted at them. And abuse that may at first be limited to a partner often grows to include abuse of the children as well. It is never better to wait.

Considering the Children

Many parents mistakenly think that children are unaware of the violence. However, researchers have found that 80 to 90 percent of the time, the kids know about the intimate violence. Even if children do not see the violence, they are affected. Hearing the fighting, seeing the bruises, and living with a suffering parent can damage children in many ways. Their reactions vary widely: some children get depressed, withdrawn, and isolated; others who witness intimate partner violence develop physical problems such as difficulty sleeping, headaches, stomach aches, and asthma. The worries that burden these children are often expressed as behavioral problems as well. Children may act out in ways that lead to poor school performance and sometimes to truancy.

It is very important to face the fact that the person who abuses you is very likely to abuse your children, if not now, then in the future. The statistics bear this out. Among households with children, anywhere from 30 to 60 percent of domestic violence situations also involve child abuse. Children from violent homes are six times more likely to commit suicide, twenty-four times more likely to commit a sexual offense, just over 50 percent more likely to abuse drugs and alcohol, and about 75 percent more likely to commit acts of violence. The risks of keeping your children in the home of an abusive partner far outweigh any possible benefit.

What to Do If You Feel You Can't Leave

If you live with a person who physically batters you, you really need to leave. That is the bottom line. Your life may truly depend on it. Even if your partner has only verbally or emotionally battered you, he or she may escalate the abuse to physical violence at some point, so it is dangerous to assume that you are safe from physical harm. (See "Planning an Escape" below to learn how to achieve a safe escape from an abusive partner.)

A safe escape involves careful planning, and you may not feel you can leave right away. As you develop your plans, take care of your general health and well-being as much as possible. Do everything you can to sustain your spirits and physical strength. Try to eat well and get enough sleep. Do things you enjoy. If you are able, try to claim some space in your home that you can call your own.

Practice being assertive. If your partner begins to verbally abuse you, gather courage and forcefully say: "Stop it." It might be easier if you rehearse doing this on your own first. Realize that one possible way to lessen the abuse is to stand up to your partner.

If you remain in an abusive household, your safety may at some point depend on the police. Do not hesitate to call 911 during an episode of abuse. Realize that abusers have killed or seriously harmed partners:

do not take a chance. If the thought of calling the police makes you feel anxious, practice beforehand what you will say. Police reports also serve as documentation of abuse (see below), and calling the police gives the message to your abuser that you are not afraid to call for help. Some women are reluctant to call the police because they think that the police will take them to jail, too. While this may have been the case in the past, these "dual arrests" (victim and abuser) are no longer the norm. Many police departments have established a system that requires an arresting officer to provide a special explanation to supervisors about why a dual arrest was made.

It is also important for you to document all episodes of abuse. This is helpful to clarify the situation for yourself, and it also provides evidence to others that abuse has been ongoing. Discuss episodes of abuse with family and friends, and let your abuser know that you have shared this information. This can be tricky, since your abuser will not want you to disclose this information. You may rightly fear that doing this will trigger a violent episode. However, your abuser will be less apt to hurt you if other people are aware of the abuse.

If you decide not to leave an abusive partner right away, you should nevertheless be prepared to escape in a crisis. Being prepared requires you to make a safety plan and to prepare an "escape bag" for yourself and your children.

Making a Safety Plan and Packing Your Safety Kit

During a violent situation, you will have a better chance at escape if you have planned ahead. A good first step is to learn about local resources by calling the National Domestic Violence Hotline at 800-799-SAFE (7233). The people who answer the phone want to help you stay safe. They can tell you where the nearest domestic violence shelter is and whether it accepts children. Knowing where a good shelter is located and how to get there will help you if you decide to escape.

You should prepare a safety kit that is ready at all times. Hide it in your own house or keep it with a trusted friend or family member. It will contain items you will need in case you make a fast escape. The abuser should not know about your plans, about the safety kit, or about how you intend to seek help. The only people who should know are people who are actually part of the plan. Here are items to put in your safety kit:

1. Spare car keys, money, a credit card or ATM card, a spare checkbook, toiletries, and a few changes of clothes for you and your children.
2. Copies of key documents, including birth certificates and social security cards for you and your children, prescription information, important legal documents, and children's immunization and school records. If you also have your abuser's social security card, put that in as well.
3. If you are fleeing with your children, it is also a good idea to include nonperishable snacks for your children.
4. A photograph of your abuser should also be in your kit. This photograph will be helpful to both police and the shelter. If a shelter employee sees someone who looks like your abuser hanging around, she can call the police. Put a photograph of your children in the kit as well.

Planning an Escape

You have your safety kit assembled and you know where the shelters are in your area. What do you do next? You need to decide how to get out. Think about how you would escape from each room in your house. Which doors lock? Which don't? Think of public places that are open 24 hours a day where you might go. If you know your partner is about to become explosive, try to get to a room that has no weapons and from which you could escape to the outside.

But what if you can't get out? And what if you can't call the police because that will make the abuser more violent? A woman in this terrible situation should confide in a friend and decide on a password or phrase that secretly communicates her danger. This will signal her friend to call the police immediately. For example, one woman said to her friend, "Have you been to that new store on Conti Street?" Her friend knew what was happening and called the police. Tell your neighbors about the violence and ask them to call the police if they hear a commotion in your home or apartment.

If you don't have to leave in a hurry, consider these other possibilities. You may want to remove pictures and other sentimental items slowly from the home so they will not be missed. Try to transfer some money from your joint accounts into an account that is in your own name. Finally, consider seeking advice from a lawyer. Many communities have free legal services for people with HIV. While domestic violence may not be their specialty, the staff there may be able to point you in the right direction to get a protective order from the municipal or family court.

What You Should Know after Your Escape

If leaving an abuser were safe and simple, everyone would do it. While the risks of staying with an abusive partner are extremely high, there are also risks associated with the time surrounding a successful escape. In fact, the risk of serious injury or homicide is highest in the first two months following separation. For this reason, unless it is absolutely necessary, women are advised not to communicate with their abusers at all right after escape.

If you have children, you may need to talk with their father once in a while. Determine a neutral location to drop off and pick up the children if they visit their father—in front of the police station, for example, or at a fast food restaurant. Do *not* let your abuser come to your home. Your abuser may do one of two things. He may say, "Hey, Baby, I love you, please come home," or he may try to hurt you. Remember that you left for a good reason. This abusive partner is the same person, and he will undoubtedly return to old behavior patterns unless he accepts that he is an abuser and is truly motivated to change. Be very careful, especially for the first few months after leaving.

When you successfully leave your abuser, you may feel wonderful. However, some women can experience post-traumatic stress disorder or clinical depression and not fully realize it. If you become very anxious or sad, or have other feelings described in chapter 16, you should seek help. Some women find themselves feeling numb, without emotion, and they isolate themselves from friends and family. This too can be a symptom of post-traumatic stress disorder.

Recognizing the abuse is the first step toward taking control of your life. Every action you take from that point forward to protect or distance yourself from your abuser is another step toward freedom and peace of mind. In addition to seeking professional help from a mental health provider, take comfort, if you can, from your friends and family. Taking control of your life is the most important thing you can do for your children and yourself.

KEY POINTS

1. *Intimate partner abuse is one partner mistreating another. The abuser's goal is to control the abused. A checklist is included in this chapter to help you determine if you are being abused.*

2. *Women may stay with abusers for several different reasons, including lack of self-confidence, wanting to believe her partner loves her, lack of resources, and concern about separating children from their father.*

3. *Children are usually aware of intimate partner violence.*

4. *Children living in an environment in which abuse is occurring are more likely to commit suicide, commit a sexual offense, use drugs and alcohol, and commit acts of violence.*

5. *If you are unable to leave an abusive situation at this time, you can practice being assertive, document episodes of abuse, discuss what is happening with friends and family and let your partner know they are aware, and prepare an escape plan.*

6. *If you plan to escape, have a safety kit hidden and plan how you will get out and where you will stay.*

7. *After your escape, do not let your abuser come to your home.*

Resources

The following national and state resources can help you find local shelters and hotlines:

National Office for National Coalition against Domestic Violence
 PO Box 18749
 Denver, CO 80128
 303-839-1852

State Coalitions against Domestic Violence

Alabama
 PO Box 4762
 Montgomery, AL 36101
 205-832-4842

Alaska
 130 Seward Street, Room 501
 Juneau, AK 99801
 907-586-3650

Arizona
 100 West Camelback #109
 Phoenix, AZ 85103
 800-782-6400, 602-279-2900

Arkansas
 7509 Cantrell Road, Suite 213
 Little Rock, AR 72207
 501-663-4668

California (Central/Northern)
 619 13th Street, Suite I
 Modesto, CA 95354
 209-524-1888

California (Southern)
 PO Box 5036
 Santa Monica, CA 90405
 213-655-6098

Colorado
 PO Box 18902
 Denver, CO 80218
 303-573-9018

Connecticut
 135 Broad Street
 Hartford, CT 06105
 203-534-5890

Delaware
 507 Philadelphia Pike
 Wilmington, DE 19809-2177
 302-762-6110

District of Columbia
 PO Box 76069
 Washington, DC 20013
 202-783-5332

Florida
 1521-A Killearn Center Boulevard
 Tallahassee, FL 32308
 800-500-1119, 904-668-6862

Georgia
 250 Georgia Avenue, SE
 Suite 308
 Atlanta, GA 30312
 800-643-1212, 404-524-3847

Hawaii
 98-939 Moanalua Road
 Aiea, HI 96701
 808-486-5072

Idaho
200 North 4th, Suite 10
Boise, ID 83702
208-384-0419

Illinois
937 South Fourth Street
Springfield, IL 62703
217-789-2830

Indiana
2511 East 46th Street, Suite N-3
Indianapolis, IN 46205
317-543-3908

Iowa
Lucas Building, First Floor
Des Moines, IA 50319
515-281-7284

Kansas
820 SE Quincy, #416B
Topeka, KS 66612
913-232-9784

Kentucky
PO Box 356
Frankfort, KY 40602
502-875-4132

Louisiana
PO Box 3053
Hammond, LA 70404
504-542-4446

Maine
PO Box 89
Winterport, ME 04496
207-941-1194

Maryland
11501 Georgia Avenue, #403
Silver Spring, MD 20902
301-942-0900

Massachusetts
210 Commercial Street, 3rd Floor
Boston, MA 02109
617-248-0922

Michigan
PO Box 16009
Lansing, MI 48901
517-484-2924

Mississippi
PO Box 333
Biloxi, MS 39533
601-436-3809

Missouri
331 Madison
Jefferson City, MO 65101
314-634-4161

Montana
1236 North 28th Street, #103
Billings, MT 59101
406-256-6334

Nebraska
315 South 9th Street, #18
Lincoln, NE 68508
402-476-6256
or

Nebraska Domestic Violence Sexual
Assault Coalition
825 M Street, Suite 404
Lincoln, NE 68508
402-476-6256

Nevada
2100 Capurro Way, Suite E
Sparks, NV 89431
800-500-1556, 702-358-1171

New Hampshire
PO Box 353
Concord, NH 03302
800-852-3388, 603-224-8893

New Jersey
2620 Whitehorse Hamilton
Square Road
Trenton, NJ 08690-2718
800-572-7233, 609-584-8107

New Mexico
PO Box 25363
Albuquerque, NM 87125
800-773-3645, 505-246-9240

New York
Women's Building
79 Central Avenue
Albany, NY 12206
800-942-6906 (English),
800-942-6908 (Spanish),
518-432-4864

North Carolina
PO Box 51875
Durham, NC 27717-1875
919-956-9124

North Dakota
418 East Rosser Avenue, #320
Bismarck, ND 58501
800-472-2911, 701-255-6240

Ohio
4041 North High Street, #101
and
PO Box 15673
Columbus, OH 43215
614-221-1255

Oklahoma
2200 Classen Boulevard, #1300

Oklahoma City, OK 73106
800-522-9054, 405-557-1210

Oregon
520 NW Davis, Suite 310
Portland, OR 97209
503-223-7411

Pennsylvania
6400 Flank Drive, #1300
Harrisburg, PA 17112
800-932-4632, 717-545-6400

Puerto Rico
Calle San Francisco 151–153
Viejo San Juan
San Juan, Puerto Rico 00905
809-722-2907

Rhode Island
422 Post Road, #101
Warwick, RI 02888
800-434-8100, 401-467-9940

South Carolina
PO Box 7776
Columbia, SC 29202-7776
803-254-3699

South Dakota
3220 South Highway 281
Aberdeen, SD 57401
605-225-5122

Tennessee
PO Box 120972
Nashville, TN 37212-0972
800-356-6767, 615-327-0805

Texas
8701 North Mopac, #450
Austin, TX 78759
512-794-1133

Utah
120 North 200 West, 2nd Floor
Salt Lake City, UT 84103
801-538-4100

Vermont
PO Box 405
Montpelier, VT 05601
802-223-1302

Virginia
2850 Sandy Bay Road, #101
Williamsburg, VA 23185
800-838-8238, 804-221-0990

Washington
200 W Street, Suite B
Tumwater, WA 98501
800-562-6025, 206-352-4029

West Virginia
PO Box 85
Sutton, WV 26601
304-765-2250

Wisconsin
1400 East Washington Avenue,
#103
Madison, WI 53703
608-255-0539

Wyoming
341 East E Street, #135A
Casper, WY 82601
307-235-2814

US Virgin Islands
8 Kongens Gade
St. Thomas, VI 00802
809-776-3966
and
PO Box 2734
Christiansted
St. Croix, VI 00822
809-773-9272

National Programs

National Domestic Violence Hotline
800-799-SAFE (7233)
TDD 800-787-3224

Battered Women's Justice Project
4032 Chicago Avenue South
Minneapolis, MN 55407
800-903-0111

Center for the Prevention of Sexual
and Domestic Violence
2400 N. 45th Street #10
Seattle, WA 98103
206-634-1903

Domestic Abuse Project
204 West Franklin Avenue
Minneapolis, MN 55404
612-874-7063

Family Violence Prevention Fund
383 Rhode Island Street,
Suite 304
San Francisco, CA 94103-5133
415-252-8900

Family Violence and Sexual Assault
Institute
1310 Clinic Drive
Tyler, TX 75701
903-595-6600

National Council on Child Abuse
and Family Violence
1155 Connecticut Avenue NW,
Suite 400
Washington, DC 20036
800-222-2000
202-429-6695

National Victim Center
2111 Wilson Boulevard, Suite 300
Arlington, VA 22201
800-FYI-CALL

National Council on Child Abuse
and Family Violence
1155 Connecticut Avenue NW,
Suite 400
Washington, DC 20036
202-429-6695
800-422-4453 (child abuse
questions)
800-537-2238 (spouse/partner
abuse questions)
800-221-2681 (counseling)

National Organization for
Victim Assistance
1757 Park Road NW
Washington, DC 20010
202-232-6682 (counseling and
business)
800-879-6682 (information and
referrals)

Parents Without Partners
401 Michigan Avenue
Chicago, IL 60611
312-644-6610

Rape Crisis Center Hotline
Washington, DC
202-333-7273
(This number will provide access to
a national directory that will provide
information about organizations in
your area.)

WOMAN, Inc.
333 Valencia Street, Suite 251
San Francisco, CA 94103
415-864-4722 (for lesbians in
violent relationships)

Women of Color Task Force Against
Domestic Violence
PO Box 1743
Aurora, CO 80040
303-696-9196

Programs for Abusers

Duluth Domestic Abuse
Intervention Project
206 West Fourth St.
Duluth, MN 55806
218-722-4134

Oakland Men's Project
1203 Preservation Park Way,
Suite 200
Oakland, CA 94612
510-835-2433

Abusive Men Exploring New
Directions (AMEND)
777 Grant St., Suite 600

Denver, CO 80203
303-832-6363

EMERGE: Counseling and
Education to Stop Male Violence
2380 Massachusetts Ave.,
Suite 101
Cambridge, MA 02140
617-547-9879

National Organization for Changing
Men/Brother Peace Raven
7314 Manchester, 2nd Floor
St. Louis, MO 63143
314-645-2075

Legal Resources

National Center for Women and
Family Law
  799 Broadway, Suite 402
  New York, NY 10003
  212-674-8200

National Clearinghouse for the
Defense of Battered Women
  125 S. 9th Street
  Philadelphia, PA 19107
  215-351-0010

The American Academy of
Matrimonial Lawyers
  150 N. Michigan Avenue,
    Suite 2040

Chicago, IL 60601
312-263-6477

Center for Battered Women's
Legal Services
  105 Chambers Street
  New York, NY 10007
  212-434-2277

NOW Legal Defense and Education
Fund
  99 Hudson Street, 12th Floor
  New York, NY 11968
  516-283-4809

Child Custody and Support Services

Child Custody Evaluation Services
of Philadelphia
  PO Box 202
  Glenside, PA 19038
  215-576-0177

The Joint Custody Association
  10606 Wilkins Avenue
  Los Angeles, CA 90024
  213-475-5352

The Association for Children for
Enforcement of Support
  723 Phillips Avenue, Suite J
  Toledo, OH 43612
  800-537-7072

Children of Divorce and Separation
  PO Box A
  Glenside, PA 19038
  800-366-8786

The Children's Foundation
  725 15th Street NW, Suite 505

Washington, DC 20005
202-347-3300

Children's Rights Council
  220 I Street NE
  Washington, DC 20002
  202-547-6227

Find Dad
  800-729-6667
A private collection agency that will
charge a percentage of the support
if collected. There is no fee if they
fail to collect.

Grandparents United for Children's
Rights
  137 Larkin Street
  Madison, WI 53705
  608-238-8751

Mothers Without Custody
  PO Box 27418
  Houston, TX 77227
  800-457-6962

16

Managing Your Feelings

How do you know if you are depressed, and what should you do about it?

What are the treatments for anxiety or nervous conditions?

What can you do if you are having trouble sleeping?

Depression

Depression is very common. Between 15 percent and 40 percent of people with HIV suffer from an episode of depression. In general, women are more likely than men to have depression, so it is not surprising that up to 60 percent of women with HIV seen in clinics have been diagnosed with depression at least once. Depressed people tend to be sad or "blue." If you are depressed, you may be unable to enjoy activities that previously gave you pleasure. Feeling sick or guilty and having a low energy level may be a result of depression and not a symptom of the HIV disease. If you are severely depressed, you may feel helpless or full of despair. Other symptoms of depression that you may experience are listed in table 16.1.

A depressed person may be more likely to do things that are harmful to her own health, such as practicing unsafe sex or using drugs or alcohol. If you are depressed, you might decide not to go to clinic or

Table 16.1
Symptoms of Depression

1. Difficulty sleeping, possibly waking up many times during the night or waking up early in the morning
2. Sleeping all the time
3. Decreased interest or pleasure in all or nearly all activities, including activities that you enjoyed before
4. Loss of energy
5. Change in appetite (eating either too much or too little) and change in weight (either gain or loss)
6. Poor concentration and memory
7. Feeling guilty or worthless (low self-esteem)
8. Difficulty functioning and making decisions
9. Hearing voices or believing part of the body is dead
10. Thoughts of death or suicide
11. Crying spells
12. Feeling hopeless

not to take your HIV treatments because you feel you don't care about anything. Not surprisingly, researchers have found that depression increases the risk of death among women with HIV. It is very important to avoid major depression. If you recognize the symptoms of early depression, you will be able to seek medical care before the situation becomes severe (see table 16.1).

Treatments for depression can be very successful. Your primary health care provider can often provide helpful advice, medications, or a referral to a mental health provider such as a psychologist (Ph.D.), psychiatrist (M.D.), or licensed clinical social worker (L.C.S.W.). Your primary care provider or mental health provider may recommend counseling or medication or a combination of counseling and medication. More than 80 percent of depressed patients find symptom relief from at least one medication. Dosage information for several antidepressant medications is listed in table 16.2.

Table 16.2
Antidepressant Brand and Generic Names and Standard Doses

Brand name	Generic name	Dose
Pamelor	nortriptyline	50–150 mg at bedtime
Norpramin	desipramine	50–200 mg at bedtime
Tofranil	imipramine	100–300 mg at bedtime
Elavil	amitriptyline	100–300 mg at bedtime
Anafranil	clomipramine	100–200 mg at bedtime
Sinequan	doxepin	150–250 mg at bedtime
Prozac	fluoxetine	20 mg in the morning
Zoloft	sertraline	50–150 mg in the morning
Celexa	citalopram	20–60 mg in the morning
Paxil	paroxetine	20–40 mg at bedtime
Luvox	fluvoxamine	150–250 mg at bedtime
Effexor	venlafaxine	75–300 mg in the morning
Remeron	mirtazapine	15–45 mg at bedtime
Serzone	nefazodone	300–400 mg in divided doses
Desyrel	trazodone	200–600 mg at bedtime
Wellbutrin	buproprion	150–400 mg/day in divided doses

In addition to relieving depression, antidepressant medications may bring other welcome side effects (see table 16.3). Antidepressants can also help with other disorders, including chronic pain, trouble sleeping, and nervous or anxiety problems. Wellbutrin (also called Zyban) has also been shown to decrease nicotine craving among people who are trying to stop smoking.

Antidepressant medications can also have unwanted side effects, however. Tricyclic antidepressants can cause a dry mouth, difficulty urinating, dizziness when getting up, blurry vision, and heart problems. Other antidepressants may have the unwelcome side effects of nausea, restlessness, weight gain, and decreased sexual arousal. (Wellbutrin is one treatment that does not have any sexual side effects.) Serzone has recently been associated with liver failure. Ask your primary care provider about the possible side effects and benefits of any medicine you are considering.

Another area of concern is the possible interactions between mental health medications and HIV treatments. You should be sure that both your mental health provider and your primary care provider know about every medication you are taking. Some mental health and HIV medications interact because they are broken down in the body by the same enzymes. These enzymes can only process so much medication at

Table 16.3
Favorable Side Effects of Antidepressants and Interactions
with HIV Treatments

Antidepressant (brand name)	Favorable side effects	HIV treatments that interact
Tricyclic antidepressants	promotes sleep, weight gain*; decreases diarrhea	Norvir and Kaletra**
Pamelor		
Norpramin		
Tofranil		
Elavil		
Anafanil		
Sinequan		
Other antidepressants	differs by treatment	differs by treatment
Prozac	may increase energy	nnRTIs and PIs***
Zoloft		Norvir**
Celexa		Norvir**
Paxil	may help with sleep	Norvir**
Luvox	may help with sleep	nnRTIs and PIs***
Effexor		Norvir**
Remeron	may help with sleep, weight gain*	
Serzone	may help with sleep	Sustiva and Crixivan
Desyrel	may help with sleep	Norvir**
Wellbutrin	may increase energy	Norvir**

* Weight gain may be an unwelcome side effect for some people.
** There is less concern about interactions with low doses of Norvir (100–400 mg a day). Norvir may increase the level of Wellbutrin and increase the risk for seizures.
*** nnRTI = non-nucleoside reverse transcriptase inhibitors; PIs = protease inhibitors

a time. If they become overloaded, blood levels of the interacting medicines can be increased or decreased away from their recommended doses. In some cases, drugs known to interact can still be taken together if they are managed with caution. If the blood levels of your medicines change substantially, however, the medications should not be given together. Be especially alert for potential interactions with the HIV drug called Norvir, which at high doses (of 600 mg twice daily) has a tendency to interact with other medications. Potential interactions between antidepressants and HIV treatments are also listed in table 16.3.

Can HIV treatments make your depression worse? In general, the answer is no. However, one treatment, Sustiva, can affect your nervous system and does have the rare side effect of either causing depression or making your depression worse. If you take Sustiva and feel worse, it is important to let both your primary care and mental health providers know.

St. John's wort is an herbal remedy that has been marketed for depression. It is available in health food stores without a prescription. However, there is a significant interaction between this herb and the powerful class of HIV medications called protease inhibitors. (These medications are discussed in chapter 6.) Because St. John's wort decreases the levels of the protease inhibitors, it is not a good idea to take St. John's wort when you are taking protease inhibitors.

If you start taking antidepressant medication, a follow-up appointment should be made for two weeks later. Your health care provider will check to see whether your mood has improved and whether you are experiencing unwanted side effects. It may take six to eight weeks before your spirits rise. Tell your primary care provider or mental health provider if you don't think the medications are working. Changes can be made in the type or dose of medication, and sometimes a second medication is added for a time. A good goal to shoot for is feeling 80 percent like your old self—that is, the medicine should make you feel 80 percent as good as you felt before the depression began.

Even after your mood improves, it is important to stay in touch with your mental health provider, because the course of depression may be chronic and you may have a relapse. About a third of patients experience a second depressive episode within one year after stopping treatment, and more than half will have another episode at some later point in their lives. People tend to take the medications only until they feel better and then quit. This is not a good idea. Some medications can be dangerous if you stop taking them "cold turkey." The abrupt change can trigger an immediate relapse into severe depression. Before you stop taking an antidepressant, discuss your plans with your provider so you can follow a safe plan for gradually discontinuing the medication and then stopping.

Anxiety Disorders ("Nerve Problems")

People with HIV do not appear to be at higher risk for most anxiety disorders or "nerve problems" than other people. A couple of conditions deserve mentioning, however, because they are fairly common—so you'll want to be aware of them. One common anxiety disorder is known as "panic attacks." People who suffer from panic attacks experience the sudden sensation that a disaster is looming or that danger is very near. These frightening feelings may occur rarely or frequently, and they are often accompanied by a rapid heartbeat and difficulty breathing. Other symptoms may include chills or hot flashes, a choking sensation, dizziness, fear of dying or of losing control, nausea, numbness or tingling, sweating, and trembling. Panic attacks are very common; up to 30 percent of all adults experience a panic attack at some time in their lives. It is important to recognize the nature of a panic attack, because the symptoms may easily be mistaken for a medical problem.

Another common anxiety disorder is "post-traumatic stress disorder," or PTSD. As its name suggests, this disorder occurs among those who survive severely traumatic events. After some delay, the person "relives" the traumatic event and then struggles to block further thoughts about it. Yet recurring dreams and nightmares may persist. People with PTSD experience extreme stress at any reminder of the traumatic event and may even feel guilty or personally responsible for it.

Certain scenarios (for example, coming into contact with someone who abused you) can potentially trigger the post-traumatic distress and anxiety. A person with PTSD will feel as if she is having a panic attack: her heart will race and her blood pressure will rise. She will try everything to avoid reminders of the traumatic experience. Women who have a past or current history of abuse may suffer from PTSD. Studies of women with HIV have shown that up to 33 percent were victims of abuse during their lifetimes. (Chapter 15 explores the topic of abuse.)

Many substances, such as caffeine (which is found in coffee, tea, and many soft drinks), nicotine, alcohol, marijuana, amphetamines, and cocaine, can affect your nervous system and make you feel anxious. You may feel more anxious if you start using one of these substances. On the other hand, if you regularly use a substance and then suddenly do without it, you may feel more anxious because you are going through withdrawal. If you feel nervous, one of the first things to do is to decrease—and ideally eliminate—use of any of the above substances. See chapter 14 for additional information on addiction and substance use.

Various treatments are used to relieve anxiety disorders. Psychotherapy, which involves counseling with a trained mental health provider, can be very effective. Medications known as anxiolytics are also frequently prescribed for anxiety (examples are listed in table 16.4). Benzodiazepines, such as Valium, are a common group of medications that can help people relax. However, you should realize that your body will become accustomed to these strong drugs and that you may experience unpleasant withdrawal symptoms if you stop taking them without slowly decreasing the dose. The person who prescribes benzodiazepines for you should closely monitor any changes in your dose, and should help you with the process of discontinuation if you wish to stop taking them. There can also be potential interactions between anti-anxiety medications and HIV treatments. Norvir is the main HIV treatment that your mental health provider should monitor carefully for interactions. Interactions are listed in table 16.4.

Table 16.4

Medications Used to Treat Anxiety and Sleep Disorders

Brand name	Generic name	Daily dose
*Selected benzodiazepines marketed for anxiety disorders**		
Ativan	lorazepam	1–10 mg in divided doses
Klonopin	clonazepam	0.25–4 mg in divided doses
Serax	oxazepam	10–30 mg in divided doses
Tranxene	clorazepate dipotassium	15–60 mg in divided doses
Valium	diazepam	2–10 mg in divided doses
Xanax	alprazolam	0.25–4 mg in divided doses
Selected serotonin (a brain transmitter) reuptake inhibitors		
Prozac**	fluoxetine	20 mg in morning to maximum
Sarafem**		40 mg in morning + 40 mg at noon
Effexor	venlafaxine	75–300 mg in the morning
Paxil	paroxetine	20–60 mg in the morning
Zoloft	sertraline	25–200 mg once daily
Other anxiolytics		
Wellbutrin	bupropion	150–400 mg daily in divided doses
Serzone	nefazodone	200–600 mg daily in divided doses
Risperdal	risperidone	2–6 mg daily
*Non-benzodiazepine medications marketed only for sleep disorders**		
Ambien	zolpidem	5–10 mg at bedtime
Sonata	zaleplon	10–20 mg at bedtime

* Selected benzodiazepines marketed solely for sleep disorders include Dalmane (flurazepam), Doral (quazepam), Prosom (estazolam), and Restoril (temazepam).
** Prozac and Sarafem are the same medication.

Trouble Sleeping

Twenty to forty percent of adults have sleep disorders. Trouble sleeping—or insomnia—occurs more frequently in women and in older individuals. People can have insomnia for many reasons. Life stresses, illness, hospitalizations, and pain can all cause insomnia, as can uncomfortable sleeping arrangements or a restless or snoring bed partner.

Caffeine, nicotine, and alcohol can act as stimulants and cause trouble sleeping. In addition to tea and coffee, many sodas contain caffeine— some contain a lot. Depression and anxiety can also interfere with good sleep.

The usual treatments for insomnia are benzodiazepines (as discussed in the preceding section). The most common ones prescribed for sleeping difficulties are Dalmane (flurazepam) and Restoril (temazepam). Ambien (zolpidem) and Sonata (zaleplon) are not benzodiazepines, but they work in a similar manner and are only marketed for treatment of insomnia.

As mentioned in the previous section, benzodiazepines pose a slight risk of physical dependence even if taken only at bedtime for sleep. You may have even more trouble sleeping if you stop taking a benzodiazepine treatment that your body has grown accustomed to. This is also true for Ambien and Sonata. The main side effect of benzodiazepines, Ambien, and Sonata is daytime sleepiness, particularly if you take any of these medications at high doses. For these reasons, it is not a good idea to start on a sleeping pill unless you really need to. Suggestions to help you sleep without medications are listed in table 16.5; table 16.6 provides additional information on medications.

Table 16.5
Strategies for Getting a Better Night's Sleep

- Seek medical advice. You may have an underlying medical problem that is causing your insomnia and that can be treated.
- Wake up and go to bed at the same time every day. Don't sleep late on weekends.
- Use the bed only to sleep, not to read or watch television.
- Stop consuming caffeine, especially after lunchtime.
- Use medication to help you sleep only on the advice of and with a prescription from your mental health or medical provider.
- Do not exercise before going to bed.
- Do not eat in the two hours before bedtime.

Table 16.6

Potential Interactions between Norvir and Some Medications
Used to Treat Anxiety or Sleep Disorders

Norvir increases levels of:	Norvir may decrease levels of:
Xanax	Ativan
Valium	Serax
Dalmane	Restoril
Klonopin	
Ambien	
Sonata	

Note: The medication names given are brand names. In general, medications listed above may still be cautiously used with Norvir. There is less concern about interactions with low doses of Norvir (100–400 mg/day).

KEY POINTS

1. Depression is very common and can respond well to treatment with counseling and medications.

2. Treatment is available for several anxiety (or nervous) conditions and may consist of counseling and medications.

3. Many women have trouble sleeping; following some simple recommendations can be helpful. Medications should be reserved as a last resort.

Resources

1. Depression Awareness, Recognition, and Treatment program of the National Institute of Mental Health at www.nimh.nih.gov/publicat/index.cfm

2. National Depressive and Manic Depressive Association at www.ndmda.org

3. National Foundation for Depressive Illness at www.depression.org

4. National Mental Health Association at www.nmha.org/ccd

5. Psychology Information Online at www.psychologyinfo.com/depression

Chronic Pain, Palliative Care, and Hospice

*Does taking opioid medications to relieve pain lead
to addiction?*

How is nerve pain treated?

How are bone and muscle pain treated?

How are headaches treated?

What are the side effects of common pain medications?

What is palliative care and hospice?

HIV and Pain

Pain, like pleasure, can take many forms. A pinch feels different from a cramp, which feels different from an ache, which feels different from a burn, and so on. Sometimes pain goes along with rewarding work, such as childbirth or exercise. And often pain serves to protect us: if we didn't feel the pain of a cut, we wouldn't know we needed to wash the wound and protect it from infection. So we know pain is important and natural and complicated. Of course we also know that pain hurts. What feels better than swift and effective pain relief?

In the past, many doctors and nurses worried that if they freely treated their patients' pain, then their patients would become addicted to the prescribed pain medications. However, research has shown that addiction very rarely happens under these circumstances. As a result, medical students are now taught not to withhold pain medications but rather to recognize and treat pain in the same knowledgeable and determined way they treat other medical problems.

Different kinds of pain demand different treatments. This chapter reviews the best approaches for easing the more common types of pain experienced by people with HIV. We begin with medications and, later in the chapter, turn to other methods for treating pain.

Most people with HIV experience pain at some point. Surveys have shown that 40 to 60 percent of people with HIV/AIDS have told their providers about pain, and over 80 percent of very ill AIDS patients suffer with pain. The pain can be caused by HIV itself, by HIV treatments, or by other problems unrelated to HIV. If you have chronic pain, you may also feel extremely tired and experience sleep problems, depression, and anxiety. You may not realize how much the pain is affecting your well-being until it is adequately controlled—and then your whole quality of life may suddenly improve.

Many studies have shown that women experience more pain than men. This may be due to hormonal differences, or it may simply mean that women are more willing to describe their pain to health care providers. Yet despite this finding, women appear to be less well treated than men for their painful symptoms.

Specific painful conditions can be diagnosed by physical examination or laboratory testing and generally receive prompt treatment. For example, problems like shingles (discussed in chapter 4) and mouth ulcers are visible and known to be painful, and providers do not hesitate to prescribe treatment for pain relief. However, pain that is not obviously connected to a physical finding or test result often receives less effective treatment. In these cases, health care providers must rely on each patient's description of her pain—and this can lead to variable pain management.

If you have pain that is poorly controlled, we suggest you keep a daily pain diary to show to your health care provider. In addition to recording how much pain you have, record how the pain limits your activities. For example, you may not be able to drive or walk any distance some days. In your pain diary, grade the severity of your pain throughout the day on a scale of zero (no pain) to ten (the worst pain you can imagine). Report these numbers to your nurse or primary care provider. A numerical scale is a good way to describe how much you hurt. In fact, doctors and hospitals often ask patients to describe their pain on a scale of zero to ten. Instead of saying "I've been in a lot of pain lately," you will communicate more useful information if you say, "I've noticed from keeping a daily diary that my pain is mild, around a 1 or 2 when I first wake up, but then it gets worse through the mornings and gets up to a 7 or 8 by lunchtime, and I can't concentrate at work in the afternoons." This information will help your primary care provider prescribe the right medicines at the right doses to get you through the day without suffering.

It is important for both you and your provider to know that it is very rare for people treated for pain to become addicted to prescription *opioids* (a term that refers to drugs derived from the opium poppy as well as to chemically similar synthetic drugs). Morphine is an example of an opioid. The term *narcotic* also refers to opioid drugs but is used in the context of describing morphine-like drugs that have the potential for abuse. The general term for any medicine that reduces pain is *analgesic.*

If you receive regular prescriptions for high doses of an opioid medication, you will probably develop a physical dependence on the drug. However, *this is different from addiction.* Physical dependence means that if you suddenly stop taking the drug you may have withdrawal symptoms. Addiction, on the other hand, involves more than withdrawal symptoms. It involves a mental preoccupation with obtaining more opioids despite adequate pain control. (Drug addiction and alcohol dependence are explored at length in chapter 14.)

Potential barriers to receiving adequate pain medication are:

• Lack of patient and provider knowledge about pain and pain control

- Little or poor communication about pain between you and your health care team
- Fear of addiction

Although you may not be able to remove all of these barriers, we hope this chapter will help improve communication between you and your health care team, as well as provide reassurance about the perceived risk for addiction.

Categories of Physical Pain

Physical pain is generally grouped into three major categories: nerve pain (called *neuropathy*); muscle and bone pain; and visceral pain, which refers to pain of the internal organs. However, not all pain easily fits into one of these categories. (For example, how would you classify the terrible pain of migraine headaches?) Still, these categories do help, because they identify the main sources of pain, which in turn helps to direct treatment. (Headaches are not included in any of these categories and are discussed separately, below.)

A person's description of her own pain is extremely important for diagnosing its origin. Nerve pain, for example, is often described as a tingling or pin-pricking sensation, or as burning or numbness. Other types of pain are not as easy to describe. Your health care provider may push you for more specific words: is it a *shooting* pain or a *throbbing* pain? Is it a *crushing* sensation or a *sharp* pain? Is it a *dull ache?* Is it a *stabbing* pain or a *wooden* feeling? Having an accurate description of the quality, location, duration, and intensity of your pain will help your health care provider find the best pain medication for you.

Medications for Nerve Pain

A number of specific non-opioid medications work very well for nerve pain. In fact, drugs that are used to treat seizures have been found to relieve nerve pain very well. Neurontin (also called gabapentin) is generally the first medication to try. Neurontin has minimal side effects. To achieve good pain relief, moderate doses of over 1,800 mg/day are often required. Your health care provider should recommend that you gradually increase your daily dose until you find good pain relief or until you reach the maximum recommended daily dose of 5,000 mg/day. If this maximum dose fails to control your pain, then a different class of medication, called *tricyclic antidepressants*, is well worth trying. Elavil (amitriptyline) is the tricyclic drug most commonly prescribed for nerve pain. (For further discussion of tricyclic medications and their possible side effects, see chapter 16.)

Zostrix, or capsaicin, and lidoderm patches are topical analgesics that can help with the discomfort caused from shingles or zoster. It can also relieve nerve pain if it is rubbed on the soles of your feet. If all of the non-opioid medications listed above still fail to control your pain, then it is appropriate to turn to opioids.

Although pain can often be controlled, numbness rarely responds to any medication. Numbness can be dangerous because the absence of feeling can cause sores or cuts to go unnoticed and then become infected. If your feet are numb, it is very important to examine them every day and to feel their surfaces, looking for blisters or cuts. People with numbness in their feet should always wear professionally fitted protective shoes and should have their feet examined by a podiatrist or other health care provider on a regular basis.

Medications for Bone and Muscle Pain

The grocery store can provide the best treatment for arthritis, muscle aches, or other related bone and muscle pain. Non-steroidal anti-inflammatory drugs, or NSAIDs, work extremely well for these disorders. Look for Motrin, Advil, Aleve, or for the generic ibuprofen. These medicines, along with several prescription NSAIDs, work by decreasing the inflammation that causes bone and muscle pain. Opioids, on the other hand, work by making you less aware of your pain.

If you have chronic bone or muscle pain, you should take NSAIDs around the clock, every 8 to 12 hours. However, if you have stomach ulcers or kidney problems, then it is not a good idea to take continuous NSAIDs, and chronic opioids may be the best treatment for you.

Medications for Visceral Pain

Conditions due to visceral pain are less common than those due to nerve pain or bone and muscle pain. Visceral pain results from illness of internal organs. For example, pancreatitis causes visceral pain because it results from an inflamed pancreas. If it is mild, visceral pain is best managed with Tylenol, aspirin, or NSAIDs, but if it is severe, as with pancreatitis, then opioid drugs are the right choice.

Pain Severity, Drug Dosages, and Precautions

In addition to considering the source of your pain, health care providers should also pay close attention to the severity of your pain. For mild pain, the World Health Organization recommends aspirin, Tylenol, or NSAIDs. For moderate pain, an opioid in addition to aspirin or Tylenol will generally work. People with chronic severe pain should receive a long-acting opioid. These are general guidelines. Table 17.1 summarizes the treatment options for nerve pain, bone and muscle pain, and visceral pain.

If you and your provider decide that it is time to try a long-acting opioid, you should also receive a short-acting opioid for "breakthrough" pain. Initially, the short-acting opioid may be a relatively mild opioid combined with Tylenol or aspirin. Some brand name drugs that offer this combination are Darvocet, Darvon, Lorcet, Lortab, Percocet, Percodan, Talwin, Tylox, Vicodin, and Tylenol 2, Tylenol 3, or Tylenol 4. If your pain is still not controlled by these combination medicines, you may need a more potent opioid such as short-acting morphine.

There is no maximum dose of "pure" opioid medications, such as morphine, but there *is* a maximum dose of Tylenol or aspirin. Therefore it is important to tell your health care provider if you are finding that you need to take six or more of your combined opioid/Tylenol or

Table 17.1
Treatment Options for Nerve Pain, Bone and Muscle Pain, and Visceral Pain

HIV-Related Nerve Pain
　First choice
　1. Neurontin (gabapentin)
　2. Other selected antiseizure medications
　3. Selected tricyclic antidepressant medications
　Second choice
　1. Zostrix cream (capsaicin)
　2. Opioids*

Bone and Muscle Pain
　First choice: NSAIDs (non-steroidal anti-inflammatory drugs)
　Second choice: Opioids*

Visceral (or Internal Organ) Pain
　1. Tylenol, aspirin, or NSAIDs for mild pain
　2. Opioids for more severe pain*

* If the pain is mild, weaker opioids, sometimes taken with aspirin or Tylenol, can be tried first. Long-acting, more potent opioids are used to treat more severe pain.

opioid/aspirin medication every day to control your pain. To prevent overdose of Tylenol or aspirin, your provider should discuss the possibility of adding a long-acting opioid to decrease your need for the short-acting combined opioid/Tylenol or opioid/aspirin.

If you have chronic pain syndrome, ideally you want to be on a regimen that takes care of the pain before it occurs or becomes severe. You do not want to wait until you are uncomfortable to take the pain medication. If you try to be stoic and endure the pain, you may be constantly miserable. The most effective treatment regimens are dosed and scheduled to help people avoid severe pain at all times.

If you have liver problems or are infected with hepatitis C, you should avoid NSAIDs and high doses of Tylenol. You can take the "pure" opioids, which include all the long-acting opioids listed in table 17.2. Short-acting "pure" opioids include Ultram (tramadol), Roxinal

Table 17.2
Long-Acting Opioids

Brand name	Generic name	Advantages	Disadvantages
Duragesic	Fentanyl	Skin patch; medication goes directly into bloodstream and needs no liver metabolism	Takes 18 hours to work, so generally need a short-acting opioid to treat breakthrough pain; works best for people with enough fat tissue
Dolophine	Methadone	Long half-life	Possible drug interactions with certain HIV treatments; associated stigma
Oxycontin	Oxycodone		High street value, associated stigma
MS Contin	Morphine		

(morphine elixir), and Oxyir or Oxyfast oral concentrate (oxycodone). If you are older or have kidney problems, certain medications may be poor choices for you. Older people are very sensitive to tricyclic antidepressants and should only receive very low doses. And people with kidney problems or stomach ulcers should avoid NSAIDs.

Headaches

If you do not suffer from chronic or recurrent headaches, you probably know someone who does. Headache is a very common pain syndrome that does not fit into one of the three pain categories discussed above. If you or someone you know experiences a sudden onset of headache or a headache that keeps getting worse, it is appropriate to seek evaluation from a primary care provider. Headaches can have a variety of causes, including certain HIV-related complications. The most common types of headache are migraine headaches and tension headaches (also called muscle contraction headaches).

Migraine headaches are often accompanied by a variety of other symptoms including mood changes, visual changes, nausea, and diarrhea. Migraine pain is classically described as "throbbing," and a migraine headache is often felt on only one side of the head. People with chronic tension-type headaches generally have very frequent headaches—more than fifteen a month—and describe their pain as a mild dull ache involving the whole head. There are no other associated symptoms as found with migraines.

The best way to treat headaches is quickly, taking pain medication as soon as you feel the headache coming on. Do not wait until you have a severe headache before reaching for your medicine. Certain types of headaches can be *prevented* with medication. Preventive medications are taken chronically rather than in quick response to an oncoming headache. Table 17.3 lists both the immediate and the preventive treatments recommended for migraine and tension headaches.

With the exception of Ultram (tramadol), chronic opioid medications are generally not prescribed for recurrent headaches. And Ultram is not recommended for people who have a personal history of opioid addiction because it has been associated with seizures if taken at a higher than recommended dose. People taking certain medications that may interact with Ultram and people with seizure histories are also at higher risk for this side effect.

Side Effects of NSAIDs and Opioids

Though non-steroidal anti-inflammatory drugs (NSAIDs) are sold over the counter under a variety of brand names, these drugs are not for everyone. NSAIDs can cause upset stomach and even stomach ulcers if taken often. People with known stomach ulcers should avoid these medications altogether. To decrease the risk of upset stomach, NSAIDs should be taken with food. In addition, anyone with a history of kidney problems should stay away from NSAIDs, which have sometimes caused kidney problems when taken chronically. People with asthma may suffer asthma attacks after taking aspirin and other NSAIDs. NSAIDs can also make it more difficult for blood to clot; for

Table 17.3
Selected Treatments for Migraine and Tension Headaches

Migraine Headaches

Immediate treatment

1. NSAIDs (non-steroidal anti-inflammatory drugs)
2. Imitrex (sumatriptan)
3. Ergotamine*
4. Cafergot* (ergotamine plus caffeine)
5. Midrin**

Preventive treatments***

1. Beta-blockers (such as Inderal, also called propranolol)
2. Calcium channel blockers (such as Calan, also called verapamil)
3. Tricyclic antidepressants
4. Selected antiseizure medications

Tension Headaches

Immediate treatment

1. NSAIDs (non-steroidal anti-inflammatory drugs)
2. Ultram
3. Midrin**

Preventive treatment: Tricyclic antidepressants

---

* Ergot drugs, such as ergotamine and Cafergot, may interact with certain HIV treatments, such as protease inhibitors. Ergot drugs should not be taken during pregnancy.

** Combination of a sympathomimetic medication, a sedative, and Tylenol.

*** Listed medications are the most common preventive therapies available, but they are not the only ones available.

this reason, anyone who is planning to visit the dentist or have a surgical procedure should avoid NSAIDs for 48 hours prior to the visit or procedure.

The side effects of opioids are quite different. The one side effect that everyone taking opioids will experience is constipation, and this side effect will persist for as long as you are taking the opioids. Therefore health care providers will prescribe stool softeners along with any prescription for opioids. If you start taking opioids and stool softeners and still do not have a bowel movement after two days, let your provider know, because you may need additional treatment for your constipation.

Nausea is also a relatively common side effect experienced when people first start taking opioids. If you feel nauseated, you will probably be given the option of changing the opioid or of taking it with an anti-nausea medication. Although opioids used for pain usually do not make people feel "high," they can make people feel "funny," sleepy, or confused during the first few days of treatment, but this side effect should go away. If these symptoms are severe, your provider may want to try a different pain regimen. When people first start taking opioid medications, they usually sleep more. This can be a good thing. Let your body rest, because you probably need the sleep.

As described above, people who take long-acting opioid medications are likely to become physically dependent on them. It is therefore important that prescriptions be filled in a timely manner, because running out of pills will lead to unpleasant withdrawal symptoms. Only certain pharmacies, such as hospital pharmacies, routinely stock the more potent long-acting opioids. If you run out of your medications on a Friday, you may not be able to get your prescription filled until Monday, and that can set you up for a bad weekend of pain and withdrawal symptoms described in chapter 14.

Treating Pain in People Addicted to Drugs

People who have a personal history of heroin or other opioid drug addiction may require higher doses of opioids to control their pain. This makes sense, because chronic opioid use can lead to drug tolerance. Pain management experts have developed formulas for adjusting the recommended doses of opioid medications for patients with opioid tolerance. Recall that there is no maximum dose for pure opioids, and sometimes high doses are necessary to control the pain of a person with a history of addiction.

However, it also makes sense first to try nonaddictive medications in people with a known tendency to drug addiction. This does *not* mean that opioids should be withheld when they are needed, but rather that primary care providers should discuss their concerns with patients and perhaps set certain restrictions on their opioid prescribing that will serve as safeguards against backsliding into renewed drug addiction. A common example of such restriction-setting is a "pain management contract." The three primary points agreed to in these contracts are:

1. Patient's agreement to have urine and blood screened periodically.
2. Patient's agreement to keep scheduled appointments and receive care from additional providers such as mental health professionals or other specialists.
3. Patient's agreement to fill prescriptions at only one pharmacy by one designated provider.

Other Therapies for Pain

Nonmedication therapies used instead of or along with medications can be very useful in relieving pain. These methods sometimes work in place of medication, and sometimes they reduce the amount of medication a person needs to take. They are particularly helpful to people who for whatever reason cannot tolerate pain medication. Listed below are a variety of techniques that have been shown to relieve pain:

- Healing therapeutic touch
- Hot or cold applications
- Deep breathing
- Massage
- Physical therapy
- Music and imagery
- Laughter and humor therapy
- Relaxation and stress-management programs
- Water therapy (such as a relaxing bath or pool exercises)

- Meditation (including prayer, yoga, tai chi, and soothing thoughts)
- Transcutaneous electrical nerve stimulation, or TENS (TENS devices deliver mild electrical stimulation and can be very effective in treating nerve pain)
- Acupuncture
- Nerve blocks (performed by an anesthesiologist)

Palliative and Hospice Care

Palliative care helps people feel better but does not cure them. To offer palliation is to relieve unpleasant symptoms, to diminish pain, and to provide comfort. People with HIV may require palliative care at any time. Some health care providers specialize in palliative care and may be available for consultation at your primary care clinic or hospital. Hospice is a specific palliative care service for people with advanced HIV disease who need additional supports and services above and beyond those provided by traditional home care.

The goal of hospice is to make very ill people feel as strong and comfortable as possible. Hospice can provide services in a person's own home, in a hospital, in a nursing home, or in any other residential facility. People who receive hospice care have decided in advance that they do not want aggressive lifesaving measures to be taken in the event that they are found unresponsive. They do not want to be put on breathing machines, for example. If you are interested in entering into hospice care or receiving hospice services, you must identify another person who will work with hospice to take care of you. (Hospice care can be given in your own home.) Hospice teams include doctors, nurses, social workers, and pastoral care providers of different faiths. The team is expertly trained to treat pain, ease symptoms, and provide emotional support. They are also usually on call 24 hours a day to offer the following skills and services:

1. Treatment of pain or other distressing symptoms
2. Nonjudgmental spiritual care and counseling for patient and family

3. Assistance with bathing and personal care
4. Emotional support
5. Respite care for patient and family
6. End-of-life planning, preparation, and counseling
7. Skilled nursing care
8. Specialized nursing on-call around the clock
9. Bereavement support for one full year after death for loved ones

Whether pain is physical or psychic, it deserves serious treatment. Fortunately, the field of pain management has made tremendous advances in the past decade. Pain, which was once considered a necessary price of illness or injury, is now aggressively relieved. Many hospitals even have specialized "pain teams" made up of pain management experts who consult with other specialists to help ease a patient's suffering.

KEY POINTS

1. People who take opioids for pain control rarely become addicted to these medications.

2. Neuropathy—or nerve pain—is treated with the drug Neurontin (gabapentin) and other anti-seizure medications, selected tricyclic antidepressant medications, Zostrix cream (capsaicin), and opioids.

3. Bone pain and muscle pain are treated with NSAIDs and opioids.

4. People with severe pain syndromes should receive long-acting opioids along with shorter-acting medication for "break-through" pain.

5. Immediate treatments for migraine headaches include NSAIDs, Imitrex (sumatriptan), Ergot medications, and Midrin; for tension-type headaches, treatments include NSAIDs, Ultram (tramadol), and Midrin.

6. For most people, the major side effects of NSAIDs are upset stomach and kidney problems. For people with asthma, NSAIDs may make breathing more difficult.

7. *The major side effects of opioids are constipation, nausea, and drowsiness.*

8. *Hospice is a palliative care service in which very ill people receive care from experts in the field of pain management.*

Resources
Growth House Search Engine at www.growthhouse.org/search.htm (a database for end-of-life issues).

18

Planning for the Future

Does HIV affect women and men differently?

Who is eligible for assistance through the social service system?

What is a living will?

Who takes care of children when a parent cannot?

Thinking about the Future

One of the first thoughts that comes to people's minds when they find out they are HIV infected is "How long do I have to live?" Today, thanks to a whole range of potent new treatment options, people with HIV are living, not dying. Even people who are very sick with AIDS-related complications when they learn about their HIV have been able to begin treatment and watch their lives turn around. HIV is no longer a disease of hopelessness. Because these phenomenal treatments have only been available since 1995, it is difficult to estimate life spans for people taking the medications, but we have every reason to expect that people who maintain very low viral loads can live as long as people without HIV.

During the early days of the HIV epidemic, women were not recognized as a population at risk and therefore were not routinely screened. As a consequence, many women with HIV did not receive the medical attention they needed until their disease had progressed, and this late recognition made it seem as though the virus worked more quickly in women than in men. Now, however, we realize that this is not the case. Because today women are often diagnosed early (in part because all pregnant women are screened for HIV), it has become clear that HIV causes women and men to become sick at the same rate. While women appear to have a lower CD4 cell count at a given viral load than men at the same viral load, the rate of CD4 cell drop over time does not differ by sex. (Chapter 3 explores this topic in detail.) In the United States, HIV no longer is allowed to progress without treatment either in women or in men.

Disability and Assistance Programs

Anyone—whether they have HIV or not—can suddenly become disabled. It is therefore important to learn about the social service system and how to navigate it should you need to. People with AIDS-defining complications of their HIV (described in chapter 4) are generally eligible for disability coverage; people with HIV who have a low CD4 count but no HIV-related symptoms usually are not. The social service system determines payments based on true inability to work. If you cannot work because you are tired, weak, and have difficulty concentrating, then you should apply for disability. If you have talked to your primary care provider in advance about these symptoms, and your limitations have been documented in your medical records, you will have a better chance of being approved for disability. If you are denied disability coverage, you can appeal the decision. If an appeal becomes necessary, it is a good idea to have your primary care provider review your chart to make sure that the nature of your disability has been well documented.

There are different types of disability incomes. Two types from the social security system include Social Security Disability Income (SSDI) and Supplemental Security Income (SSI). If you have worked in the past but are unable to work now, you may qualify for disability income.

If your job does not provide this benefit, Social Security may give you SSDI. Whether you qualify depends on whether or not you have paid into the Social Security system for a specific amount of time and whether the Social Security Administration finds you disabled.

SSI is different from SSDI. Whether you qualify for SSI and how much you would potentially receive depends on your means. Your means are whatever you own, combined with whatever income you receive, including SSDI payments. People with greater need receive greater assistance. If you need financial assistance to care for your children, you may also qualify for Aid to Families with Dependent Children (AFDC). The amount of AFDC money you receive depends on the number of children you have and on your income. AFDC money can only be used for your children's needs.

General Public Assistance (GPA) is offered through the states and differs from one state to the next. As with other assistance programs, the amount of support you qualify for depends on your means. Some clinics employ social workers and case managers to assist clients with disability applications. If your clinic does not offer these services and you are applying without help, keep a careful record of the name of every person you talk to and what you talked about. It is a good idea to keep all these notes together in a single spiral notebook or folder so that all your information is in one place when the time comes to apply at the Social Security office. You will also need to bring proof of your identity, address, and date of birth, along with your Social Security card and proof of income, assets, medical expenses, living expenses, and dependents.

The application process can often be challenging, frustrating, and prolonged. Sometimes people who receive disability income later find the strength to work part-time and are then faced with the choice of forfeiting their disability benefit if they demonstrate the ability to work at all. This can be quite aggravating for people who need disability income but who also want to work as much as they can. Because the process is complicated, it is always a good idea to talk with your primary care provider before you apply. In addition, seek the help of a case manager or social worker if that is an option in your area.

Living Wills and Advance Directives
(Wishes Regarding Resuscitation)

While nobody enjoys thinking about end-of-life planning, it is a task we all need to face. Even people with no medical problems at all should consider what they would want to happen to them if they were to become catastrophically ill. What if you were in a serious accident? What if your heart stopped beating? Would you want emergency resuscitation? These important but unpleasant questions can be answered in a legal document called a "living will." If you do not have a living will, also known as "advance directives," very personal medical decisions will likely be made for you by strangers. Emergency room doctors and other members of the health care team would always rather know for sure what each patient wishes. When an injured or ill person cannot clearly state her wishes in the given moment, advance directives can guide decision making in the right direction.

If a person stops breathing, then emergency personnel will put that person on a breathing machine—unless a living will makes it clear that the person did not want to be put on a respirator. If a person's heart stops beating, then emergency personnel will run a strong current of electricity through the person's body to try and restart the heart—unless a living will makes it clear that this should not be done. These dramatic medical interventions may or may not be successful, but without the written directive "do not resuscitate," or "DNR," emergency teams are obligated to try all life-saving measures available.

It makes sense (and can provide peace of mind) to take care of living-will paperwork before you are in a situation where it might become relevant. However, if you are hospitalized and have not completed a living will, you can still make your wishes known by having your primary care provider write an order in your chart stating that you do not wish to be resuscitated (if that is the case). Your primary care provider should ask you about your wishes at the time of your admission. Understand that having a living will does *not* stop you from receiving general medical treatment or from receiving treatments intended to make you more comfortable, such as pain medication or oxygen. If you do decide to make a living will, a copy of it should go in your medical chart and a copy should be given to your family.

At some point you may decide that you do not wish to ever be hospitalized. Sometimes people who have had multiple hospitalizations for HIV-related complications decide that they would rather turn to hospice care than return to a hospital. Hospice, which is described more fully in chapter 17, is a service for people with medical conditions that will not improve. Hospice nurses are experts in pain management whose goal is to make you feel as strong and comfortable as possible in your own home or in a home-like residential hospice center.

Wills and Guardianship

All adults should have written wills, and all parents should designate guardians for their children in the event that something happens to them. As with living wills, these documents will ensure that your personal wishes will be honored when it comes time to make decisions regarding your children, money, and property. If you have property and die without a will (called "dying intestate"), then the property will go to your spouse, to your children, or to your nearest living relative, depending on the laws of the state where you live.

If you have children, one of the most important things you can do for them is to decide who will take care of them if something happens to you. Your wishes can be included in your will, or you can stipulate your wishes in a separate document called a "deed of guardianship." In this deed, you can list reasons why you think a particular person should be the guardian of your children. If you die while your children are still minors, the deed will usually be filed in court and will influence the court's decision regarding guardianship.

You can also designate someone as the legal guardian of your children while you are still alive. A petition for a guardian of a minor is filed in court. The child's other parent and "interested persons" will be notified so that they have the opportunity to consent or object to your choice of guardian. If your child's other parent disputes the petition, you will have to show that the other parent is unfit. Evidence of addiction, abuse, or abandonment, or incarceration can make a parent unfit in the eyes of the law. The court will also need to approve of the guardian. When the court appoints a guardian, that person becomes the legal caretaker of the children and can receive public benefits and assistance.

Taking Control

Taking control of your life will make a difference. The legal preparations described above are only one example of the many ways to take control of your life. The more you learn about your body, about health care, about social services, and about other people in your situation, the more powerful you will be. Knowledge is power. Knowing how to take care of yourself will prolong your life and help you avoid sickness. Knowing how to work with your health care team will leave you feeling better both physically and mentally.

Reading this book is a start, but realize that new information is being released every day. You can stay informed by continuing to read new publications. Appendix 2 lists a number of AIDS organizations that can send you up-to-date publications written for people living with HIV. If you have access to a computer, you can visit hundreds of Web sites that provide clear, accurate information about HIV and other medical problems. A reference librarian in your public library can help you learn to use the Internet. Be assertive in seeking knowledge. Ask your primary care provider about anything you don't understand. It is critical to keep learning so that you can make the best possible decisions for yourself both today and into the future.

KEY POINTS

1. Men and women appear to be similarly affected by HIV.

2. If you have an AIDS-defining complication, you should be eligible for disability through the Social Service system.

3. A living will is a document that outlines your wishes regarding medical resuscitation.

4. *You can document your wishes regarding guardianship of your children in one of two ways: in a will, or in a deed of guardianship.*

Resources

The Kaiser Family Foundation (KFF) at www.kff.org provides publications about policy and the healthcare system.

19

Research Studies and Clinical Trials

How do researchers learn about how HIV infection affects women's health?

What protections are there for volunteers who participate in research studies?

What happens if a study treatment is found to pose risks?

Who has access to personal information obtained through clinical studies?

What are the advantages and disadvantages of participating in a study?

Why Volunteer for Research Studies?

Today we know a great deal about both HIV infection and HIV treatments. Our information came from volunteers who were willing to participate in research studies and clinical trials. Without carefully conducted scientific studies, we would have no way of knowing which treatments work, which treatments don't, and which should be avoided by whom. Anyone who shops in a pharmacy owes a debt of gratitude to the people who enrolled in the past studies that proved the safety and efficacy of every FDA-approved medication and medical appliance sold in the United States. By enrolling in a clinical study, you are ensuring that this progress and protection continue.

Most of the early data about HIV came from studies that enrolled few women. Although there has been an increase in the number of female study volunteers over time, most current HIV treatment studies are still enrolling more men than women. Researchers still need to enroll more women to determine if there is a sex difference in the side effects, effectiveness, or circulating blood levels of different HIV treatments. Will women yield the same findings as men? We still do not know.

For this reason, there has been a tremendous effort to encourage women's participation in studies. It is widely recognized that it is more difficult to find female study volunteers. In the past, studies often excluded women "of childbearing potential"—meaning all women who *might* get pregnant. Studies today do not have this exclusion unless there is a good medical or scientific reason. However, most studies do require that women use birth control while enrolled in the study. Some other potential barriers to participation include transportation problems and childcare responsibilities. To improve access both to health care and to study participation, many clinics now offer women assistance overcoming these two barriers.

Some women still hesitate to join studies. Despite the clear value of contributing to medical knowledge, they may worry about confidentiality or about their own safety. But there are regulations in place to protect all study volunteers by guaranteeing both confidentiality and an acceptable balance between the possible risks and benefits of participation. This chapter explains these regulations and defines a number of important terms related to clinical studies. We hope you will read this chapter with an open mind, appreciating the very important role you can play as a study volunteer. Your personal decision to join a study will make a real difference in the ability of researchers to develop better treatments for HIV.

Regulations That Protect You

Every study conducted in the United States or run by American investigators must be approved by an Institutional Review Board (IRB). Members of these boards are usually doctors, nurses, and other health care professionals. In addition, every IRB is supposed to have a member of the community on the board, someone who brings the perspective of a nonmedical person to the review process. The job of the IRB is to evaluate proposed and ongoing studies, making sure that the following considerations are appropriately managed in every case:

- First, there must be an acceptable balance between the possible risks posed to study volunteers and the possible benefits presented to them. An IRB should not approve any study that has large risk and small potential benefit.
- Second, the rights of study volunteers must be protected. If someone who is enrolled in the study wishes to leave the study, that person should still be guaranteed to receive medical treatment.
- Third, study participants must understand the possible risks posed by the study before they consent to enroll. The consent form must be clear and appropriately obtained. It should be carefully reviewed by the person considering enrollment in a comfortable setting where all questions can be fully answered.

Studies must be accepted by an approved IRB before they are allowed to begin. Every study is then continually reviewed at periodic intervals to be sure that the risk/benefit balance has not changed. Any complications or negative side effects (also called adverse events) that occur must be reported to the IRB and to other groups that are responsible for monitoring the study. If problems emerge and it appears that the possible risks are starting to outweigh the possible benefits, then the study will be shut down early.

IRBs also take great care to protect the confidentiality of study records. Generally, investigators can only collect information about volunteers that is needed for the research. They may use codes instead of individuals' names on any papers that record study results. Study records must be kept in locked locations, and there should be a plan to destroy the records at some point after the study is completed. Only study personnel who are involved with the study should have access to the records. The exception to this are certain members of those groups allowed by law to look at the records: the Food and Drug Administration (which is the government group that approves medications) and the relevant IRB itself. Representatives from these groups need to have access to the records so the study can be monitored. The FDA and the IRB make sure the study is done correctly and the rules are followed. If you are offered the chance to participate in a study, make sure that the study is approved by an IRB. Ask the study staff if you are unsure.

The FDA has been inspecting studies for the last forty years. If the study involves a medication, the FDA may come and inspect the location doing the study. The FDA may make sure that volunteers on studies have signed informed consent forms, for example, and that any treatment side effects have been noted and reported. If the FDA finds any problems, that site may not be able to continue doing studies until the problems are fixed.

In 1996 Congress passed the Health Insurance Portability and Accountability Act (HIPAA). One of the consequences of this law is that there are now many more safeguards in place to keep your health information (also called protected health information) private. In addition to signing an IRB-approved consent form to enter a study, you also now need to sign an HIPAA consent form if the study needs to use any of your protected health information.

What to Expect If You Volunteer for a Study

There are several ways you might learn about studies in which you may be eligible to participate: from your primary care provider, from other clinic personnel, or through advertising. Ideally, you should discuss the study with your primary care provider before enrolling. If you have never volunteered for a study before, your provider can go over the ad-

Table 19.1

Advantages and Disadvantages of Study Participation

Possible Advantages

1. You are helping answer the question: What is the best way to treat HIV?
2. The study may offer tests that give you extra information about your own health that may be beyond the scope of routine primary care.
3. You may gain access to treatments that are not otherwise available.
4. The study may pay for your treatments, lab tests, and provider visits.
5. Transportation to the clinic may be provided.
6. You may receive small payments for each study visit to reimburse you for transportation costs or for time lost from work.
7. You may have less waiting time for clinic visits, and you may have a wider range of available appointment times.
8. You will have the benefit of additional health personnel, such as the study nurse, who will both monitor your health and answer your questions.

Possible Disadvantages

1. You may need to delay starting treatment for a few weeks, though this should not greatly affect your health.
2. You may not know which treatment you are receiving.
3. The study may decide which HIV treatment you will receive.
4. You may need to come to the clinic more frequently than otherwise.
5. You may have more tests done than if you were not on a study.
6. Usually studies do not allow you to become pregnant.
7. You may experience side effects.
8. You may not get any benefit from the study.

vantages and disadvantages of participating. These features are summarized in table 19.1.

If you want more information about ongoing studies in your area, your primary care provider can refer you to a study nurse who can explain specific studies to you in detail. If you decide to participate in one of these studies, the nurse will ask you to sign a consent form. These forms can be several pages long. They can also be somewhat intimidating because they list every side effect that anyone on the study drug has experienced. They may also contain some difficult language. If there are words on the form that you do not confidently understand, have the nurse define them for you. Some of the more common terms you might encounter are explained later in this chapter. Table 19.2 summarizes the main features you can expect to see on a consent form.

If you are younger than 18 years of age, you will need to have a parent or guardian sign the consent form with you. If you are pregnant, your baby's father may also need to sign the form. Rules regarding the father's consent have recently changed. Now, a father's consent is only required if the research offers potential benefit to the baby but not to the mother. The father's consent is not required if there is potential benefit to the mother or if there is no direct benefit to the mother or baby but the risk of the study is minimal.

Signing a consent form does not mean that you are required to par-

Table 19.2

Information Generally Included in a Study Consent Form

1. The study title
2. Where the study is being done
3. The names and contact numbers of the people running the study
4. A description of the study and what question or questions the study is addressing
5. Possible benefits of the study
6. Possible risks of the study
7. Possible reasons why you might need to come off the study
8. Statements about your right to refuse to participate and about your right to withdraw from the study
9. A description of who will have access to your study results and of how the study will protect your confidentiality
10. Financial information regarding whether you will receive any payments and explaining who pays for medications, tests, provider visits, and possible complications
11. Places for you and a witness to sign the consent form. If you are blind, a reader can sign for you. If you are younger than 18 years, your parent or guardian will need to sign.

ticipate in the study. You can change your mind immediately after signing. If you enroll in a study and later decide to withdraw, your medications may change, but your care should not be otherwise affected. (Your treatment regimen may change because certain medicines are only available through clinical trials.)

Once you have decided to participate in a research study and have signed the consent form, you will usually have "screening" blood work done to make sure that you are an appropriate candidate for the particular study that interests you. Even if your primary care doctor has ordered blood tests for you in the recent past, the study will probably require you to have some tests repeated. It usually takes a few days for the laboratory to return your test results. If your results indicate that the particular study is not a good match for you, then the study nurse will talk with you about your options and will refer you back to your primary care provider. Otherwise, you will be ready to begin.

The study nurse will provide you with your medication, explain in detail how to take the treatments, and schedule your next appointment. You should be given a number to call during the day or evenings if you have any questions or problems. You usually need to bring all your medicines to every study visit. As discussed in chapter 6, HIV treatments can be difficult to manage. They involve several medicines, each with its own dosing schedule. Remembering to take every dose of every medicine can be a complicated task. Your study nurse may count the pills left in the bottle to help determine if you took every dose. Health care providers and patients have found this practice of "double-checking" to be very helpful. Talking about the experience of taking the medicines and actually counting out the pills allows time for you and your nurse to work together to make sure that you are getting the medicine you need and that the study's findings will be accurate. It is very important for your study nurse to know if you are having trouble taking your medications. Together, you can develop strategies to make the process easier and more successful. No one will judge you for finding it a challenge.

While research studies do *monitor* your HIV infection, study personnel do not provide primary care. If you experience any new symptoms while participating in a study, or if you are simply not feeling well, you should call your study nurse. But do not be surprised if the nurse asks you to schedule an appointment with your primary care provider. Your care will still be provided by your original health care team, but the study nurse also needs to keep track of any symptoms that may be related to the study's treatments.

Understanding the Language of Research Studies

Many people have heard of "clinical trials" or "clinical studies," but what do these terms actually mean? If you are thinking about participating in a study, it is important to understand the definitions of several terms associated with clinical research. The following section will help clarify the scientific language used to describe these studies.

Pre-clinical Trial

Pre-clinical simply means "before the clinic." New drugs are first tested in laboratories and in animals. These early studies determine a drug's major side effects; they reveal how effective the trial drug is against different organisms or HIV; and they suggest how the drug will probably be metabolized by people. Most drugs tested in pre-clinical studies never go on to be tested in humans. If an experimental drug shows serious side effects or simply does not work in animals, it does not go forward to people. However, if a new drug looks promising, the FDA grants it the status of an Investigational New Drug (IND). The drug must have an IND rating before it can be used in human studies.

Clinical Trial

All prescription medicines in the United States have been approved by the FDA. The FDA grants approval based on a drug's safety and effectiveness. How does the FDA determine whether a drug is safe and effective? With clinical trials. These trials involve human volunteers and can last anywhere from a few days to several years, depending on the nature of the drug under investigation. A clinical trial involves the pharmaceutical company making the drug, investigators who run the study, and the FDA, which oversees the process. A medication is considered experimental until the FDA licenses, or "approves" it. To participate in a clinical trial, each study volunteer has to meet certain criteria. During the course of the study, volunteers are monitored for certain outcomes, and data on these outcomes are collected to show whether the experimental treatment is working safely and effectively. Clinical trials are divided into four "phases," as described below.

Phase 1 Clinical Trial. Before a great number of volunteers can be given any experimental medication, it is necessary for researchers to determine a safe dose of the drug. This determination is made with a phase 1 clinical trial. A phase 1 trial relies on a small number of volunteers, usually about twenty people. It generally lasts only a few days or weeks and often requires that volunteers stay overnight in a research unit. During the phase 1 trial, volunteers will be started on a low dose of the investigational drug, and then the dose will be slowly raised as long as no bad side effects develop. Study volunteers will have their blood drawn at different intervals to determine the circulating drug levels over time. This testing helps show how quickly a person's body will metabolize each particular dose. Based on the drug levels and side effects, researchers can then determine the best dose to use in the next phase of the clinical trial.

Phase 2 Clinical Trial. Phase 2 clinical trials determine if a drug is effective. They are much larger than phase 1 trials and generally enroll more than one hundred volunteers. Phase 2 trials may last for several months or years. While determining a drug's effectiveness, these trials also gather additional information about side effects and dosing.

Phase 3 Clinical Trial. You may have heard the phrase "gold standard" applied to a particular medical treatment. This refers to whatever treatment approach is widely considered by specialists to be the best choice for a given medical condition. The "gold standard" is the treatment doctors prescribe first. Phase 3 clinical trials compare the investigational drug to the "gold standard" treatment for whatever condition both seek to address. Phase 3 studies are very large and may enroll over one thousand volunteers. Like phase 2 trials, phase 3 clinical trials last for months to years. For people who are interested in trying new treatments that have not yet been approved by the FDA, participating in a phase 2 or phase 3 clinical trial may allow access to the desired treatment.

Phase 4 Trial. After a drug has been approved and licensed by the FDA, pharmaceutical companies may wish to obtain additional information on its side effects or on possible new uses for the drug. Studies conducted after a drug has already been licensed by the FDA are called phase 4 trials.

New Drug Review. At the end of a phase 3 clinical trial, the pharmaceutical company that makes the investigational drug will gather all its study findings and submit them to the FDA in the form of a New Drug Application. The FDA then reviews this information and decides whether to license the experimental drug. If it does approve the medication, the FDA will not only list appropriate indications for the drug's use but will also recommend the best dose and decide which side effects require warnings.

Randomization. Things that are random happen by chance. In research studies, "randomization" of volunteers to different treatments is very important to prevent biased results. Why? Consider the following situation. Suppose you want to compare drug "A" to drug "B." If volunteers could *choose* which drug they wanted to take rather than be randomly assigned, then it might turn out that women generally choose drug A for some reason and men generally choose drug B. If 95 percent of the people taking drug A are women and 95 percent of the people taking drug B are men, then any differences found between the two groups might be due to sex differences rather than to any difference between the drugs. On the other hand, if both groups had equal numbers of men and women, then any difference found between drug A and drug B could not be due to sex difference.

Randomly assigning volunteers to different treatments prevents the sort of biased conditions described above. It works like flipping a coin: heads, you get drug A, and tails, you get drug B. Chance will decide. Randomization guarantees that the study design will be well balanced for any characteristics that might wrongly influence the study's findings.

Blinding. Studies can be "blind" or even "double blind." Blinding is another technique for eliminating bias. *Blinding* means that the person taking a medication does not know what medication she is taking. Suppose that drug A has a reputation for making people's teeth itch. If a volunteer knows she has been assigned to take drug A, she might be inclined to pay more attention to her teeth and to think they feel itchy. Do they really itch more, or is she just feeling this sensation because she expects to? Without blinding, there is no way to know. And what if her primary care provider knows she is taking drug A? Might that person be more inclined to ask specifically about that symptom? If neither the patient nor the health care provider knows which study medication is being taken, then the study is "double blinded," and is even more secure from bias. In this situation, only the pharmacist knows for sure which study volunteer is taking which drug. To achieve blinding, different medications can be made to look alike. (The method does not always work perfectly, because some side effects are very common with certain medications, and this gives them away.)

Placebo. A placebo is a pill that does not contain any medicine at all. While a placebo may look exactly like a real drug, it isn't. The "placebo effect" is when people report that their symptoms improve thanks to the placebo pill, which they believe is a real medicine. In other words, some people actually feel better simply because they believe that they are receiving treatment, even though they really are not. A "placebo-controlled trial" is designed to tell the difference between a real drug effect and a placebo effect. However, there are no placebo-controlled trials for HIV treatments, because it is already well established that HIV medications work to control the infection. Therefore, it would be unethical to give a placebo drug to a person with HIV. *Currently, all studies investigating HIV treatments compare different active medications, and never placebos.*

IN SUMMARY, well-controlled clinical trials overseen by Institutional Review Boards and by the Food and Drug Administration are responsible for all FDA-approved medications and medical appliances sold in the United States. By volunteering to participate in a clinical trial, you are helping researchers to develop new, safe, and ever more powerful treatments for the medical conditions that affect so many thousands of people in this country and around the world.

KEY POINTS

1. The only scientific way to learn about women's response to HIV infection and to HIV treatment is to have women participate in well-controlled studies.

2. Every good study is overseen by an approved Institutional Review Board, which is a committee of professionals who review the possible risks and benefits of each study.

3. Institutional Review Boards can call a stop to any study if possible risks associated with it appear to be greater than the associated benefits.

4. Test results obtained for a study are held confidential and only authorized persons can access the information.

5. You can explore possible advantages and disadvantages of study participation with your primary care provider.

Resources

1. ACTIS at www.actis.org or call 1-800-874-2572 or 1-800-243-7012 (information on completed and ongoing studies).
2. AMFAR at www.amfar.org (information on clinical trials and drug assistance programs).
3. HIV InSite Trials Search at http://never.ucsf.edu:8000/tsearch (a clinical trials database).
4. AIDS Treatment Data Network at www.aidsinfonyc.org/network (information on studies).
5. Canadian HIV Trials Network at www.hivnet.ubc.ca/ctn.html (information on studies in Canada).
6. Adult AIDS Clinical Trials Group at http://aactg.s-3.com (information on treatment studies for adults).
7. Pediatric AIDS Clinical Trials Group at www.pactg.s-3.com (information on treatment studies for pregnant women and children).

8. Terry Beirn Community Programs for Clinical Research on AIDS (CPCRA) at www.cpcra.org (information on treatment studies for adults).

9. The Bulletin of Experimental Treatments for AIDS (BETA) at www .sfaf.org/treatment or call 1-800-959-1059.

10. AIDS Clinical Trials and HIV research in women at https:// statepaips.jhsph.edu/wihs (describes the Women's Interagency HIV Study or WIHS, a long-term follow-up study of women with and without HIV).

Appendix 1

Sample Tracking Sheet for Medications, Tests, and Vaccinations
(Use as a model for how to set up your own tracking sheets)

Medication*	Dosage	Date Begun	Date Stopped	Side Effects
1.				
2.				
3.				
(etc.)				

Blood Test		Date	Results
CD4 cell count			
CD4 cell count %			
Viral load level			
Cholesterol/lipid panel			
Genotype/phenotype results**			
Other tests***			
1.			
2.			
3.			
(etc.)			

Pap smear/cervical biopsy	Date	Results

Mammogram	Date	Results

Vaccines/shots given****	Date

* List every medication, even nonprescription therapies. If a medication is stopped, note why (i.e., side effect, not working, etc.).
** Ask your primary care provider to photocopy the results, and attach them to the tracking sheet.
*** If you have any abnormal tests, record the results of these tests over time to follow the trends of the test results. Abnormal tests might include blood count (if you are anemic or have other blood count abnormalities), blood sugar testing (if you have diabetes), liver function tests (particularly if you are co-infected with a hepatitis virus), and kidney function tests.
**** If you receive Depo or birth control shots, keep a record of the dates you receive the shots.

Appendix 2

Resources for People with HIV

Note: Additional resource information on specific topics is listed at the end of selected chapters.

WEB SITES AND PHONE NUMBERS

Aegis at www.aegis.com. *General HIV information and resources.*

Centers for Disease Control National Prevention Information Network at www.cdcnpin.org or call (800) 458-5231 or (800) 243-7012.

Community AIDS Treatment Information Exchange (CATIE) at www .catie.ca.

Critical Path AIDS Project at www.critpath.org.

Johns Hopkins University AIDS Service at www.hopkins-aids.edu *or* www.hopkins-aids.edu/publications/index_pub.html. *Information on multiple topics relating to HIV.*

New York Online Access to Health (NOAH) at www.noah.cuny.edu/ about.html.

Project Inform at www.Projectinform.org. *General patient education.*

PWA Health Group at www.aidsinfonyc.org/pwahg or call (212) 255-0520.

Seattle Treatment Education Project (STEP) at www.thebody.com/ step/steppage.html or call (877) 597-STEP (7837) toll-free from the Pacific Northwest (Washington, Oregon, Idaho, Alaska, and Montana).

The Body at www.thebody.com. *Information on HIV prevention, treatment, conferences, and quality of life.*

University of California at San Francisco at www.HIVInSite/ucsf.edu. *Information on general HIV topics and treatments.*

Women Alive at www.women-alive.org or call (800) 554-4876 or (323) 965-1564.

Women Organized to Respond to Life-threatening Disease at www .womenhiv.org or call 510-986-0340.

HIV/AIDS PHONE RESOURCES

Direct AIDS Alternative Information Resources (888) 951-5433

Latino Commission on AIDS (CIEST) (212) 675-3288

National AIDS Clearinghouse (800) 458-5231

National AIDS Hotline (800) 342-2437 (Spanish) (800) 344-7432

National AIDS Treatment Advocacy Project (NATAP) (888) 26 NATAP or (212) 219-0106

National Association of People with AIDS (202) 898-0414

National Minority AIDS Council (202) 483-6622

Treatment Action Group (212) 260-0300

Glossary

Abacavir: See *Ziagen.*

Abuse: The mistreatment of one person by another. Abuse can be physical, sexual, emotional, or verbal (chapter 15).

Acquired Immune Deficiency Syndrome: See *AIDS.*

Acyclovir: See *Zovirax.*

Addiction: Addiction to drugs differs from physical dependence and is characterized by a person's extreme efforts to obtain the drug, to take the drug more frequently and at higher doses than advised by a doctor, and to spend a majority of time using the drug, recovering from its effects, and trying to obtain more. People can be addicted to prescription drugs as well as to illegal drugs. Alcoholism is a form of addiction (chapter 14).

Adefovir: See *Hepsera.*

Agenerase (also called amprenavir): A protease inhibitor HIV treatment (chapter 6).

AIDS (Acquired Immune Deficiency Syndrome): Persons are diagnosed as having AIDS if they have a CD4 cell count less than 200 or if they have a specific medical condition associated with having a CD4 cell count below 200. People with HIV infection whose CD4 counts remain above 200 and who do not have any AIDS-defining medical conditions do not have AIDS. Opportunistic or AIDS-defining medical conditions include specific infections and cancers, as well as symptoms such as extreme forgetfulness, confusion, or loss of at least 10 percent of body weight (chapter 4).

AIDS Clinical Trials Group (ACTG): A group of medical centers all over the United States that perform clinical studies. The medical centers in the group are called AIDS Clinical Trials Units (or ACTUs). The ACTG is supported by money from the National Institutes of Health (chapter 19).

Alcoholism: A form of addiction. A person suffering from alcoholism spends a majority of time consuming alcohol, recovering from the drinking, and trying to obtain more alcohol. Addiction of any form generally impairs a person's ability to work, participate well in family life, or maintain a healthy social life (chapter 14).

Aldara cream (also called imiquimod): A medication used to treat the genital warts that result from human papillomavirus (HPV) infection (chapter 7).

Alendronate: See *Fosamax.*

Alzheimer's disease: A form of severe dementia that exceeds the mild symptoms of confusion or forgetfulness often seen with normal aging.

Amenorrhea: An interruption of menstrual cycles for at least six months (chapter 12).

Amitriptyline: See *Elavil.*

Amphotericin: A medication given intravenously for treatment of serious fungal or yeast infections.

Amprenavir: See *Agenerase.*

Anabolic treatments: Specific hormones, including Anadrol (oxymetholone) and Oxandrin (oxandrolone). Anabolic therapies cause muscle weight gain and are related to testosterone, a male sex hormone (chapter 4).

Anemia: A low red blood cell count (chapter 4).

Anergy: The inability to mount an immune reaction to an antigen. A person with tuberculosis who has a very low CD4 cell count may be unable to show a skin reaction to the standard PPD test that screens for tuberculosis; this person would be considered "anergic" (chapter 4).

Antibiotic: Medications that fight bacteria. Antibiotics do not work against viruses. Examples include penicillin, Bactrim, and Zithromax.

Antibody: Proteins made by the body to fight infections.

Antigen: Proteins that come from organisms outside a person's own body. People make antibodies to foreign antigens.

Antiretroviral experienced: Persons who have taken antiretrovirals or HIV treatments before (chapter 6).

Antiretroviral naive: Persons who have never taken any antiretrovirals or HIV treatments (chapter 6).

Antiretrovirals: A class of medications designed to treat retroviruses like HIV (chapter 6).

ASCUS: See *Atypical squamous cells of undetermined significance.*

Atazanavir: See *Reyataz.*

Atorvastatin: See *Lipitor.*

Atovaquone: See *Mepron.*

Atypical squamous cells of undetermined significance (ASCUS): A Pap smear test result often caused by infection with human papillomavirus (HPV), an infection that can lead to cervical cell changes and sometimes to cervical cancer (chapter 9).

Azithromycin: See *Zithromax.*

AZT: See *Retrovir.*

Bacterial vaginosis: A condition thought to result from a change in the type of bacteria (or an overgrowth of certain bacteria) that live in the vagina. It is often associated with a fishy odor and vaginal discharge (chapter 8).

Bactrim (also called trimethoprim/sulfamethoxazole): An antibiotic used both to treat and to prevent certain bacterial infections. It is the medication of choice to prevent and treat *Pneumocystis carinii* pneumonia (PCP) (chapter 4).

Benzodiazepines: A group of medications commonly prescribed for anxiety, difficulty sleeping, and seizures. Valium is an example of a benzodiazepine. These drugs make people feel more relaxed, but they can also cause sleepiness, confusion, and physical dependence, which can lead to withdrawal symptoms if the drugs are abruptly stopped (chapter 16).

Biaxin (also called clarithromycin): An antibiotic prescribed for various bacterial infections. It is also used to prevent and treat *Myco-bacterium avium-intracellulare* complex (MAC), an opportunistic infection that affects people with low CD4 cell counts (chapter 4).

Biopsy: A small tissue sample that is sent to a laboratory for disease diagnosis.

Bisphosphonates: A class of medications used to treat osteoporosis and strengthen bones. Fosamax is an example of a bisphosphonate (chapter 13).

Blinding: A study designed to prevent the volunteer from knowing which medication he or she is taking. A double-blinded study also prevents the primary care provider from knowing which study medication is being given to the volunteer. (Only the pharmacist filling the prescription will know for sure.) The purpose of blinded studies is to prevent biased outcomes (chapter 19).

Blood cell count: Monitoring of blood cells. Red blood cells transport oxygen, white blood cells are part of the immune system, and platelets help blood clot. A low red blood cell count is called *anemia,* a low white blood cell count is called *leukopenia,* and a low platelet count is called *thrombocytopenia.* HIV treatments can affect blood cell counts in different ways, and anyone taking these medications needs frequent blood monitoring.

Boosted protease inhibitor: Adding a low dose of Norvir (100 to 400 mg) to your protease inhibitor regimen to increase the blood levels of the specific protease inhibitor (chapter 6).

Bronchoscopy: A procedure involving an illuminated scope that allows specialized doctors to examine the inside of a patient's lungs and to collect samples of secretions or tissue for laboratory analysis.

Candida: See *Candida esophagitis.*

Candida esophagitis: A yeast infection that can spread from the mouth down into the esophagus and cause pain or difficulty swallowing (chapter 4). See also *Thrush.*

CAT scan (computerized tomography scan): A special type of X-ray that provides a three-dimensional view of the body. A person undergoing a CAT scan often receives an injection of contrast material before the X-ray is taken, since it shows up on the final images and can clarify certain structures. A CAT scan is a painless procedure that requires the person to lie in a tubular chamber that is open on one end. A CAT scan can reveal infections, abnormal growths, bleeding, and other problems.

Catapres (also called clonidine): A blood pressure medicine that may help reduce hot flashes in women going through menopause (chapter 12).

CD4 cell count: CD4 cells are also called T4 cells or T-helper cells. Because HIV directly targets CD4 cells, they are the part of the immune system that is carefully monitored in people infected with HIV. The absolute CD4 cell count is used to gauge the amount of immune system damage caused by HIV (chapter 3).

Centers for Disease Control and Prevention (CDC): A federally funded institution located in Atlanta, Georgia, that monitors epidemic and other diseases. The CDC is notified about anyone who is diagnosed with AIDS. The CDC uses this information along with descriptive data such as sex and race to track the epidemic. The information collected by the CDC is used to request support for AIDS services from the federal government. Personal data are not shared with other agencies and are kept very secure.

Cerebrospinal fluid (CSF): CSF bathes the brain and spinal cord. Infection of the CSF leads to meningitis, which is diagnosed by withdrawing a CSF sample through a lumbar puncture, a procedure also known as a spinal tap.

Cervical dysplasia: Precancerous changes in the cells of the cervix, a finding that may be discovered in a Pap smear or a cervical biopsy (chapter 9).

Cervical intraepithelial neoplasia (CIN): Precancerous changes in the cells of the cervix, a finding that may be discovered in a Pap smear or a cervical biopsy (chapter 9).

Cervicitis: An infection of the cervix, a condition that sometimes causes vaginal discharge and lower abdominal pain but that sometimes causes no symptoms at all (chapter 8).

Cervix: Part of the uterus. It is shaped like a ring and connects the lower uterus to the top of the vagina.

Chemokine receptors: The entry of the virus into cells is helped by "chemokine receptors" named CCR5 and CXCR4 (chapter 6).

Chlamydia: A bacterium that frequently causes cervicitis and pelvic inflammatory disease (PID) (chapter 8).

Chronic carrier: A person who has maintained a positive hepatitis B surface antigen for at least six months (chapter 5).

Cidofovir: See *Vistide.*

Clarithromycin: See *Biaxin.*

Clinical trial: The proof of a medicine's safety and effectiveness is obtained through studies called clinical trials. A clinical trial involves many people: study volunteers, the pharmaceutical company that makes the medication, study investigators who run the trial, an Institutional Review Board that approves the study, and the Food and Drug Administration, which oversees the study's quality and safety (chapter 19).

Clonidine: See *Catapres.*

Cocktail: An informal term for the various combinations of HIV treatments that are recommended for greatest effect against HIV. They are also known as "HAART regimens" (chapter 6).

Colposcopy: An outpatient medical procedure that allows a gynecologist to see the cervix through a magnifying glass and take a biopsy from any areas that appear to have abnormal changes (chapter 9).

Combivir: A combination of Retrovir and Epivir (chapter 6).

Community Programs for Clinical Research on AIDS (CPCRA): A group of medical centers all over the United States that perform studies related to HIV and AIDS. CPCRA is supported by money from the National Institutes of Health and is a different group from the ACTG.

Cone procedure: A small surgery that may require brief hospitalization but that may spare a woman the need for a hysterectomy. With this procedure, a gynecologist cuts out the part of the cervix known to contain abnormal, precancerous cells (chapter 9).

Crixivan (also called indinavir): A protease inhibitor HIV treatment (chapter 6).

Cryptococcal meningitis: Cryptococcus is a fungus that most often goes to the brain and can cause meningitis (an infection of the lining around the spinal cord and brain). This infection is acquired by inhalation. *Cryptococcus* can also cause pneumonia or a blood infection. People with cryptococcal meningitis usually have a headache and fever and can be very ill, requiring hospitalization (chapter 4).

Cryptosporidiosis: Cryptosporidium is a parasite that can contaminate water and cause severe diarrhea (chapter 4).

Cytomegalovirus infection (CMV): An active CMV infection can cause retinitis—an inflammation of the back of the eye. Rarely, CMV can also infect the gastrointestinal tract and cause bloody diarrhea and stomach pain. If CMV infects the brain, symptoms include confusion, weakness, and even paralysis (chapter 4).

Cytovene (also called ganciclovir): A medication used to treat cytomegalovirus infections (CMV). It can be given by mouth, through the vein, or by an implant surgically placed in the eye.

d4T: See *Zerit.*

Dapsone: An antibiotic medication used to prevent and treat *Pneumocystis carinii* pneumonia (PCP) (chapter 4).

Daraprim (also called pyrimethamine): An antibiotic medication used to treat toxoplasmosis (chapter 4).

ddC: See *Hivid.*

ddI: See *Videx.*

Deed of Guardianship: A legal document that identifies the person a parent has designated to be the guardian of her or his children after the parent has died (chapter 18).

Delavirdine: See *Rescriptor.*

Dementia: The symptoms of dementia include memory loss and difficulty concentrating. HIV-related encephalitis/dementia is caused by the effect of HIV on the brain (chapter 4).

Depo shots: Short for "depoprovera," Depo shots are progestin hormone injections that are given every three months as a method of birth control. This form of contraception often causes irregular menstrual bleeding or stops the menstrual periods altogether (chapter 10).

Depoprovera: See *Depo shots.* For uses other than as birth control, depoprovera can also be given daily by mouth.

DEXA scan: The best screening test to determine bone strength is called a DEXA scan, which stands for *dual energy X-ray absorptiometry* (chapter 13).

Didanosine: See V*idex.*

Diflucan (also called fluconazole): An oral medication used to treat cryptococcal meningitis, yeast infections such as thrush, yeast vaginitis, and *Candida* esophagitis (chapter 4).

Down's syndrome: A chromosomal (or DNA) disorder that causes mild to severe mental retardation in newborns, as well as other abnormalities. Older mothers are more likely to have babies with Down's syndrome.

Ectopic pregnancy: An ectopic pregnancy results when the fertilized egg implants somewhere outside the uterus, most commonly in one of the fallopian tubes. These pregnancies do not survive and can lead to life-threatening bleeding in the mother if they are not treated. Blood tests in combination with an ultrasound study can diagnose ectopic pregnancy.

Efavirenz: See *Sustiva.*

Elavil (also called amitriptyline): A medication used to treat nerve pain (chapter 17).

ELISA test: A blood test used to screen for HIV infection (chapter 1).

Emergency contraception: Estrogen and progesterone combination medications taken within 72 hours after intercourse to prevent pregnancy (chapter 10).

Emtricitabine: See *Emtriva.*

Emtriva: (also called emtricitabine or FTC): A nucleoside reverse transcriptase inhibitor HIV treatment (chapter 6).

Endometriosis: A relatively common disorder that may cause pelvic pain. Normally, endometrial tissue lines the uterus. Women with endometriosis have additional endometrial tissue located outside the uterus (chapter 12).

Endometrium: The inside lining of the uterus (also called the womb).

Endoscopy: A procedure (usually outpatient) in which a specialist uses a narrow tubular scope with a light to see internal anatomic structures such as the esophagus, the stomach, or the rectum and colon.

Enfuvirtide: See *Fuzeon.*

Entry inhibitors: The class of drugs that block HIV cell entry is called "entry inhibitors." Entry inhibitors include attachment, chemokine receptor, and fusion inhibitors. Several under study may be available in the near future (chapter 6).

Eosinophilic folliculitis: An itchy rash that causes bumps usually all over the body (chapter 4).

Epivir (also called lamivudine or 3TC): A nucleoside reverse transcriptase inhibitor HIV treatment (chapter 6).

Epogen: See *Erythropoietin.*

Erythropoietin: The brand names for erythropoietin are Procrit and Epogen. These are treatments that stimulate the bone to produce more red blood cells. They work for anemia caused by HIV or HIV treatments. Procrit and Epogen must be injected underneath the skin, but they can be given as infrequently as once a week (chapter 4).

Esophagus: The anatomical tube connecting the mouth and the stomach.

Evista (also called raloxifene): A medication used to treat osteoporosis by strengthening the spine and hip bones. Evista is an alternative to taking hormone replacement therapy (chapter 13).

Famciclovir: See *Famvir.*

Famvir (also called famciclovir): An oral medication used to treat herpes infections, one cause of genital sores (chapter 8).

Fatigue: Extreme tiredness or lack of energy (chapter 4).

Femring: A vaginal ring that releases estrogen for hormone replacement therapy (chapter 12).

Fetal alcohol syndrome: If a mother drinks alcohol while she is pregnant, her baby may develop fetal alcohol syndrome, which can cause slower growth, a smaller head, heart problems, and severe mental retardation.

Fibrocystic breast disease: A noncancerous condition that causes breasts to feel lumpy. Women with fibrocystic breast disease do not have a higher chance of developing breast cancer (chapter 13).

Flagyl (also called metronidazole): An oral medication used to treat bacterial vaginosis and trichomonas (chapter 8).

Fluconazol: See *Diflucan.*

Follicle stimulating hormone (FSH): FSH signals the ovaries to produce estrogen. As women begin to go through menopause, their ovaries produce less estrogen and their FSH levels increase. The FSH level is a blood test used to confirm menopause (chapter 12).

Food and Drug Administration (FDA): The federal agency responsible for ensuring that medications are safe and effective. The FDA also decides whether a medication can be sold over the counter or will require a prescription.

Fortivase (also called saquinavir): A protease inhibitor HIV treatment (chapter 6). An older and weaker formulation of saquinavir is called invirase.

Fosamax (also called alendronate): A medication used to treat osteoporosis by strengthening the bones (chapter 13).

Fosamprenavir: See *Lexiva.*

Foscavir (also called foscarnet): A medication given through the vein to treat cytomegalovirus infections (CMV).

FTC: See *Emtriva.*

Fusion inhibitors: A class of HIV treatments that work by blocking the fusion (or linkage) between the envelope surrounding HIV and the cells in a person's body. The only currently available fusion inhibitor is Fuzeon (chapters 3 and 6).

Fuzeon (also called T-20 or enfuvirtide): The first fusion inhibitor HIV treatment. Fuzeon is given as shots twice daily.

Gabapentin: See *Neurontin.*

Ganciclovir: See *Cytovene.*

Gemfibrozil: See *Lopid.*

Generic name: The scientific name of a drug. Many generic drugs also have brand names.

Genital ulcer: A sore located in or around the vagina, penis, or rectum (chapter 6).

Genotype testing: Blood tests that identify viral resistance to antiretroviral treatments. The test looks for changes in the virus (called mutations) that will cause resistance to specific HIV treatments (chapter 6).

Gonorrhea: A bacterium that frequently causes cervicitis or pelvic inflammatory disease (PID) (chapter 8).

HAART: See *Highly active antiretroviral therapy.*

Hematology/oncology: A medical subspecialty that gives doctors expert training in the management of blood disorders, including cancer.

Hepatitis: Inflammation of the liver (chapter 5). Hepatitis is often caused by different viral infections, particularly hepatitis A, B, and C. Many medications, including certain HIV treatments, can also cause hepatitis. Symptoms include right upper stomach pain, nausea, vomiting, and a yellowing of the skin, called jaundice.

Hepsera (also called adefovir): A medication used to treat hepatitis B.

Herpes simplex virus: Herpes simplex virus (HSV) is a sexually transmitted disease that frequently causes genital sores. It can also cause sores elsewhere on the body (chapter 8).

High density lipoprotein (HDL) cholesterol: HDL cholesterol is good cholesterol. High HDL levels will lower a person's risk for heart disease (chapter 9).

Highly active antiretroviral therapy (HAART): A HAART regimen includes three or more anti-HIV treatments, including at least one potent therapy. The potent antiretrovirals include all of the protease inhibitors (PIs), all of the NNRTIs, and one of the RTIs (Ziagen) (chapter 6).

Hivid (also called zalcitibine or ddC): A nucleoside reverse transcriptase inhibitor HIV treatment (chapter 6).

Hormone replacement therapy (HRT): The oral estrogen and progesterone that many women take after menopause to relieve menopausal symptoms and to prevent osteoporosis (chapter 12).

Hospice: A service for people with medical conditions that will not improve, such as advanced cancer or AIDS. Hospice helps people feel as comfortable and strong as possible and is intended for people who do not want to return to the hospital. Hospice staff are experts in pain control and end-of-life issues (chapter 16).

HPV: See *Human papillomavirus.*

Human growth hormone: See *Serostim.*

Human papillomavirus (HPV): HPV infections can cause genital warts and abnormal Pap smears. There are several HPV types, and specific "high risk" types (i.e., types 16, 18, 31, 35) are associated with precancer or cancer findings (chapter 9).

Hydrea (also called hydroxyurea): A medication sometimes used along with antiretroviral regimens to make the antiretrovirals stronger. While Hydrea is not an antiretroviral treatment itself, this medicine enhances the effectiveness of antiretrovirals such as Videx (chapter 6). However, Hydrea can have bad side effects, and for this reason it is rarely used.

Hysterosalpingogram: An X-ray in which dye is first injected into the uterus and fallopian tubes so that this reproductive anatomy shows up in the X-ray images. This test can show whether the fallopian tubes are blocked, a condition that would interfere with a woman's ability to become pregnant.

Imiquimod cream: See *Aldara cream.*

Immune system: The system directly damaged by HIV infection. The immune system allows a person to fight infections of all kinds. It is a complex system made up of many different cell types, each with an important role in protecting the body from harmful bacteria, viruses, parasites, and fungus. It also helps us heal from sickness and injury (chapter 3).

Indinavir: See *Crixivan.*

Infertility: The inability to conceive a baby after a full year of regular intercourse with no contraception.

Insomnia: The inability to fall asleep easily or to stay asleep through the night (chapter 16).

Institutional Review Board (IRB): A committee that reviews clinical research studies performed by American investigators. The IRB makes sure proposed studies have an acceptable balance between risks and benefits. The IRB is also responsible for reviewing consent forms. Studies performed in the United States must be IRB approved (chapter 19).

Integrase inhibitors: A class of drugs that block the integrase enzyme essential for integrating the HIV-DNA into your chromosomes or the genetic material in your body's cells. Integrase inhibitors are a new class of drugs under study that may be available in the future (chapter 6).

Intensification: Making your regimen stronger, either by adding an HIV treatment or by making one of your HIV treatments stronger, such as boosting a PI in your regimen (chapter 6).

Interferon-alpha: see *Roferon-A* and *Intron-A.*

Intrauterine device (IUD): A birth control device that is inserted into the uterus. It works by preventing any egg from implanting in the wall of the uterus. IUDs can increase the risk for pelvic infections and should ideally be used in women at low risk for STDs.

Intron-A: A treatment for hepatitis B and C (chapter 5).

Invirase (also called saquinavir): A protease inhibitor HIV treatment. The new, stronger version of saquinavir is called Fortivase.

Isoniazid (INH): An antibiotic medication used to treat tuberculosis (chapter 4).

Jaundice: Yellowing of the eyes and skin due to increases in bilirubin levels in the blood. Bilirubin results from turnover of red blood cells through the liver. Jaundice suggests liver disease unless it is due to specific HIV treatments (Reyataz and Crixivan).

Kaletra (also called lopinavir/ritonavir): A protease inhibitor HIV treatment (chapter 6).

Kaposi's sarcoma: A type of cancer that causes purple and red skin bumps. Kaposi's sarcoma is very rare in women; however, unlike men, women with Kaposi's sarcoma often have the cancer spread throughout the body to the lungs and internal organs (chapter 4).

Lactic acidosis: A rare medication side effect probably related to nucleoside reverse transcriptase inhibitors. It causes nausea, vomiting, and stomach pain (chapter 6).

Lamivudine: See *Epivir.*

Laparoscopy: A surgical procedure that involves making a small incision into the belly button through which a narrow laparoscope can be inserted. A laparoscope is a device that allows the gynecologist to see the pelvic cavity without having to make a major incision or conduct a major surgery. In addition to normal anatomy, laparoscopy can reveal pelvic inflammatory disease, endometriosis, abnormal tissue growth, and other disorders.

Lexiva (also called fosamprenavir): A protease inhibitor HIV treatment that is a "pro-drug" of Agenerase (see chapter 6).

Lipitor (also called atorvastatin): A medication used to treat abnormal blood fat levels. It is a statin drug that has little interaction with protease inhibitor therapies (chapter 13).

Lipodystrophy: Changes in body shape and increases in blood fat and sugar levels. Lipodystrophy is more likely to occur in people who have taken HIV treatments, but the cause of lipodystrophy is unknown (chapter 6).

Loop electrosurgical excision procedure (LEEP): An outpatient procedure that burns away any cervical cells showing abnormal, precancerous changes (chapter 9).

Lopid (also called gemfibrozil): A treatment for elevated triglyceride levels (chapter 13).

Lopinavir/ritonavir: See *Kaletra.*

Low-density lipoprotein (LDL) cholesterol: LDL cholesterol, or "bad cholesterol," is a form of fat in the blood. At high levels LDL can increase a person's risk for heart disease. High LDL levels are treated with dietary changes and, if necessary, with medications (chapter 13).

Lunnelle: An injectable method of birth control. The shots contain the same hormones as oral contraceptives (chapter 10).

Lymphadenopathy: Swollen lymph nodes that can occur around the neck, under the arms, and in the groin area. Generally swollen lymph nodes due to HIV infection are not painful and do not mean the HIV infection is progressing (chapter 4).

MAC: See *Mycobacterium avium-intracellulare complex.*

Magnetic resonance imaging (MRI): An MRI is a special X-ray test that gives three-dimensional images of the interior of the body. It is the preferred test to look for problems in the head or spinal cord. When having an MRI, a person lies in a large tube and remains motionless for 30 to 60 minutes. Claustrophobia can be a problem. People who have any metal in their bodies (such as a pin from a prior surgery) cannot have an MRI done.

Marinol (also called dronabinol): A medication prescribed to treat nausea and to improve appetite. Marinol is derived from marijuana (chapter 14).

Megace (also called megestrol acetate): A hormone treatment prescribed to improve appetite. It usually causes fat weight gain (chapter 4).

Meningitis: An infection of the cerebrospinal fluid (CSF). Symptoms usually include fever, headache, and stiff neck. Meningitis can be caused by bacteria, viruses, fungi (such as *Cryptococcus*), and parasites.

Mepron (also called atovaquone): An antibiotic medication prescribed to prevent and treat *Pneumocystis carinii* pneumonia (PCP) (chapter 4).

Metronidazole: See *Flagyl.*

Microscopic: Something that can only be seen under the microscope.

Microsporidium: A parasite that can cause symptoms similar to those caused by *Cryptosporidium,* including diarrhea and upset stomach. Not everyone with microsporidiosis has symptoms.

Mirena intrauterine device: The newest IUD on the market. It also releases progestin or hormones. The progestin thickens the cervical mucus, suppresses ovarian function, and inhibits sperm movement, which enhances the effectiveness of this IUD (chapter 10).

Mutations: Changes in the structure of a virus or bacteria that can make them more resistant to medications. Mutations in HIV can produce a new strain of the virus, and treatments that used to work might not work on the new strain (chapter 6).

Myalgia: General muscle aches (chapter 4).

Mycelex (also called clotrimazole): A topical medicine used to treat fungal or yeast infections. The troche is often used to treat thrush.

Mycobacterium avium-intracellulare complex (MAC): A bacterium related to tuberculosis but not infectious to other people and the symptoms are not as severe. MAC blood infections can cause high fevers, weight loss, diarrhea, cough, and a general feeling of being sick (chapter 4).

Mycobutin (also called rifabutin): Prescribed to prevent and treat *Mycobacterium avium-intracellulare* complex (MAC) infections in people with low CD4 cell counts (chapter 4).

Narcotics: See *Opioids.*

National Institutes of Health (NIH): A federal organization that funds scientific research in the United States, including research pertaining to HIV/AIDS. The AIDS Clinical Trials Group (ACTG) and Community Programs for Clinical Research on AIDS (CPCRA) are funded by the NIH.

Nelfinavir: See *Viracept.*

Neurontin (also called gabapentin): A medication prescribed to treat nerve pain.

Neuropathy: Nerve pain or discomfort, which can take different forms. People may feel numbness, tingling, or pain in the feet and legs and possibly in the fingers and hands. Neuropathy may come and go, or it may persist (chapter 4).

Nevirapine: See *Virammune.*

Non-nucleoside reverse transcriptase inhibitors (NNRTIs): A class of HIV treatments that work by blocking specific enzymes in the HIV to keep the virus from reproducing (chapters 3 and 6).

Nonoxynol-9: A spermicide. Frequent use of nonoxynol-9 can cause vaginal irritation and even genital sores (chapter 10).

Non-progressors: People infected with HIV whose immune systems do not appear to be affected by the virus and who do not suffer from any HIV-related complications even after several years of infection.

Non-steroidal anti-inflammatory drugs (NSAIDs): Medications used to treat musculoskeletal pain and menstrual cramps. Motrin, or ibuprofen, and Aleve, or naproxen, are examples of NSAIDs.

Norplant: An implantable progestin medication used for birth control. The Norplant device implanted into a woman's arm will prevent pregnancy for five years. Norplant will cause irregular periods or might stop the woman's period altogether (chapter 10).

Norvir (also called ritonavir): A protease inhibitor HIV treatment (chapter 6).

NSAIDs: See *Non-steroidal anti-inflammatory drugs.*

Nucleoside reverse transcriptase inhibitors (RTIs): A class of HIV treatments that work by blocking the reverse transcriptase enzyme to keep the HIV from reproducing (chapters 3 and 6).

Nucleotide reverse transcriptase inhibitors (RTIs): A class of HIV treatments that differs slightly from nucleoside RTIs that work by blocking the reverse transcriptase enzyme to keep the HIV from reproducing. Viread is the only currently available nucleotide RTI (chapters 3 and 6).

NuvaRING: A vaginal ring that releases hormones for birth control (chapter 10).

Nystatin: A topical medicine used to treat fungal or yeast infections. The "swish and swallow" method is frequently used for thrush, a yeast infection of the mouth and esophagus (chapter 4).

Opioids: Heroin and prescription opioid drugs (also known as narcotics) are produced from a flower, the opium poppy. Opioid drugs are generally prescribed for pain. When managed by an experienced health care provider, prescription opioids may lead to physical dependence but rarely to addiction (chapter 17).

Opportunistic processes: Certain medical conditions occur only in people who have experienced damage to their immune systems. These are termed opportunistic processes. Examples include specific infections, cancers, and symptoms such as extreme weight loss or for-getfulness (chapter 4).

Oral candidiasis: See *Thrush.*

Oral contraceptive pills (OCPs): Birth control pills taken once daily. Each pill generally combines estrogen and progesterone (chapter 10).

Oral glucose tolerance test: This simple blood test examines how well the body metabolizes sugar. A person is asked to drink a sugary liquid and then have her blood drawn for testing one hour later. People with diabetes have high blood sugars and may require medication.

Ortho-evra: A birth control patch that contains the same hormones as those found in oral contraceptives (chapter 10).

Osteonecrosis: Dying bone. Osteonecrosis is not related to osteoporosis, and having one of these conditions does not increase the risk for the other. The risk of osteonecrosis may be increased with certain HIV treatments (chapter 13).

Osteoporosis: Thinning bones. Having thin bones increases a person's risk of fracture, especially in the back and hip bones (chapter 13).

Ovulation: The ovary's release of an egg into the fallopian tube.

Palliative care: Care that aims to make a person feel more comfortable emotionally, physically, and spiritually but does not aim to cure dis-ease. Hospice service provides palliative care (chapter 17).

Pancreatitis: An inflammation of the pancreas. It can result from exces-sive alcohol consumption, from viral infections, from gallstones, and from certain medications (such as the HIV treatment Videx). Symp-toms of pancreatitis include stomach pain, nausea, and vomiting.

Papanicolaou (Pap) smear: An outpatient procedure performed during a pelvic examination. A small brush or swab is guided around the cervix to collect cells for evaluation under the microscope. The cells are spread onto a glass slide and sent to a laboratory (chapter 9).

PCP: See *Pneumocystis carinii pneumonia.*

PCR: See *Polymerase chain reaction test.*

Pegasys: A pegylated interferon medication used to treat hepatitis C. Pe-gylated interferon lasts longer than standard interferon and needs to be given only once each week (chapter 5).

Peg-intron: A pegylated interferon medication used to treat hepatitis C. Pegylated interferon lasts longer than standard interferon and needs to be given only once each week (chapter 5).

Pegylated interferon-alpha: See *Peg-intron* and *Pegasys.*

Pelvic inflammatory disease (PID): PID refers to an infection of the uterus and fallopian tubes. Symptoms include fever, lower abdominal pain, and vaginal discharge (chapter 8).

Pentam (also called pentamidine): A medication used to prevent and treat *Pneumocystis carinii* pneumonia (PCP) (chapter 4). Pentam may be inhaled or administered to a person through a vein (intravenously).

Pentamidine: See *Pentam.*

Phase 1 clinical trial: Before being released to the general public, all medications are first tested in a multiphase process of clinical trials. The first phase—phase 1—evaluates the safety and appropriate dosing of a medication under investigation (chapter 19).

Phase 2 clinical trial: As part of the research that precedes a new drug's approval for sale, phase 2 clinical trials assess the medication's effectiveness and potential side effects (chapter 19).

Phase 3 clinical trial: As part of the research that precedes a new drug's approval for sale, phase 3 clinical trials compare the investigational drug to the "gold standard," or accepted medication for a particular medical condition. Phase 3 studies are very large and may enroll more than one thousand volunteers and last for months to years (chapter 19).

Phase 4 trial: After a drug is licensed, a pharmaceutical company may wish to obtain additional information on side effects or new indications for use. Studies done after the drug has been licensed by the FDA are called phase 4 studies (chapter 19).

Phenotype tests: Blood tests that can check for resistance to antiretroviral treatments. Phenotype testing determines whether HIV will grow in containers with HIV treatments (chapter 6).

Phytoestrogens: Hormones contained in many plants, fruits, and vegetables, such as soy and legumes. They may relieve some symptoms associated with menopause and are an alternative to hormonal replacement therapy (chapter 12).

PID: See *Pelvic inflammatory disease.*

Placebo: A pill that does not contain any active medication but that can be useful in research studies. Clinical trials involving the treatment of HIV do not use placebos.

Pneumococcus: The most common bacterial cause of pneumonia. There is a vaccine that can help protect against this infection (chapter 4).

Pneumocystis carinii pneumonia (PCP): An opportunistic infection that can affect people with very low CD4 cell counts. Symptoms of PCP infection include fever, shortness of breath, and cough. The pneumonia may be mild or very serious. Antibiotics can be taken to prevent PCP infection in people with low CD4 cell counts (chapter 4).

Pneumonia: Infection of the lung. The symptoms generally include fever, shortness of breath, and cough. Pneumonia can be serious and may require hospitalization. It is caused by various organisms. If the pneumonia is caused by bacteria, the infection may be referred to as bacterial pneumonia. *Pneumocystis carinii* is another common organism that can cause pneumonia among persons with HIV (chapter 4).

Polymerase chain reaction (PCR) test: This laboratory test evaluates genetic material and can be used to detect the presence of HIV in a person's blood. PCR is not routinely used to screen adults, but it is often used to check whether newborn infants are HIV-infected (chapter 1).

Polyurethane: A substance used to make condoms; polyurethane condoms are recommended for people who are allergic to latex condoms (chapter 7).

Post-traumatic stress disorder (PTSD): An anxiety disorder that affects people after they experience a traumatic event. Physical or emotional abuse can lead to PTSD (chapter 16).

Pravachol (also called pravastatin): A medication used to reduce blood fat levels. It is a statin drug that has less interaction with protease inhibitor therapies for HIV than do other statin drugs (chapter 13).

Pravastatin: See *Pravachol.*

Pre-clinical trial: A new drug is first studied in test tubes and in animals. These early studies determine the drug's major side effects, effectiveness, and metabolism (chapter 19).

Prempro: A hormone replacement therapy used to treat menopausal symptoms or to prevent osteoporosis. Prempro combines estrogen and progesterone into one pill that is taken daily (chapter 12).

Primary care provider: A primary care provider is a health care professional who oversees a person's medical care and who generally provides the first evaluation and treatment of new symptoms. This person may be a doctor, a nurse practitioner, or a physician's assistant. Primary care providers often refer their patients to medical specialists as needed, but they continue to manage their patients' general health needs (chapter 2).

Procrit: See *Erythropoietin.*

Prophylaxis: Treatment given to prevent disease, not to treat a disease.

Protease inhibitors (PIs): A class of HIV treatments that work by blocking the protease enzyme to keep the virus from reproducing (chapters 3 and 6).

PTSD: See *Post-traumatic stress disorder.*

Pulmonary: A medical subspecialty that evaluates and treats lung problems.

Pyrazinamide (PZA): An antibiotic medication prescribed to treat tuberculosis (chapter 4).

Pyrimethamine: See *Daraprim.*

Raloxifene: See *Evista.*

Randomization: In clinical trials involving study volunteers, the process called randomization is used to prevent biased outcomes. Randomization means assigning volunteers to different treatments based on chance. This guarantees that the study will be well balanced for any characteristics that might influence outcomes (chapter 19).

Rebetrol (also called ribavirin): A treatment for hepatitis C (chapter 5).

Rescriptor (also called delavirdine): A non-nucleotide reverse transcriptase inhibitor HIV treatment (chapter 6).

Retinitis: Inflammation of the back of the eye.

Retrovir (also called zidovudine or AZT): A nucleoside reverse transcriptase inhibitor HIV treatment (chapter 6).

Reyataz (also called atazanavir): A protease inhibitor HIV treatment (chapter 6).

Rifabutin: See *Mycobutin.*

Ribavirin: See *Rebetrol.*

Rifadin (also called rifampin): An antibiotic medication prescribed to treat tuberculosis (chapter 4).

Rifampin: See *Rifadin.*

Ritonavir: See *Norvir.*

Roferon-A (also called interferon-alpha): A treatment for hepatitis B and hepatitis C (chapter 5).

Saquinavir: See *Fortivase and Invirase.*

Safe sex: Sex that poses no risk of HIV transmission because there is no exposure to a partner's blood, vaginal secretions, or semen (chapter 7).

Safer sex: Sex that carries a very slight risk for HIV transmission. An example of safer sex would be intercourse with the use of condoms (chapter 7).

Seborrheic dermatitis: A rash with dry, flaky skin. It occurs most often around the nose and between the eyebrows (chapter 4).

Selective serotonin reuptake inhibitors (SSRIs): A class of medication used to treat depression and selected anxiety disorders (chapter 16).

Seroconversion: When a person who has been infected with HIV has made enough antibodies to the virus to yield a positive result on an HIV blood test (chapters 1 and 3).

Serostim (also called human growth hormone): An injectable treatment to counter weight loss (chapter 4).

Shingles: A rash caused by herpes zoster, the chicken pox virus. The rash of shingles is usually limited to a single area of the body and looks like a patch of small blisters (chapter 4).

SIL: See *Squamous intraepithelial lesions.*

Skin test: Generally refers to the test that looks for exposure to tuberculosis. It involves sticking a tiny needle just under the skin and injecting a purified protein from tuberculosis. Most people who have been previously exposed to tuberculosis will form a wide red bump at the injection site, in reaction to the protein. This response is considered a "positive" result. People with significant immune system damage may not respond, however. This inability to mount a response is called *anergy* (chapter 4).

Social Security Disability Income (SSDI): Financial assistance from the Social Security Administration for people who have paid into the Social Security system for a specific amount of time and who become disabled (chapter 18).

Spermicide: A method of birth control that works by killing sperm. Spermicides may be gels, foams, or creams. While spermicide may give some protection against certain sexually transmitted diseases, it will not protect a person from HIV (chapters 7 and 10).

Spina bifida: A baby with spina bifida is born with incomplete closure of the backbone. This birth defect can be minor, or it can cause severe neurologic damage.

Spinal tap (also called a lumbar puncture): The procedure used to obtain a sample of cerebrospinal fluid to look for meningitis. A very thin needle is passed between the backbones in the lower spine. The procedure can be done in an outpatient clinic and usually takes about 30 minutes.

Squamous intraepithelial lesions (SIL): Precancerous changes in cells of the cervix. This finding is one possible result of a Pap smear (chapter 9).

SSDI: See *Social Security Disability Income.*

SSRIs: See *Selective serotonin reuptake inhibitors.*

St. John's wort: An alternative treatment marketed for depression that is often available in health food stores. This treatment has been shown to have significant interactions with certain protease inhibitors and is not recommended for people taking HIV treatments (chapter 16).

Statins: A group of medications used to treat abnormal blood fat levels. Some statins may interact with protease inhibitors (chapter 13).

Stavudine: See *Zerit.*

Structured Treatment Interruption (STI): A strategy in which HIV treatments are stopped if a person meets certain criteria (chapter 6).

Supplemental Security Income (SSI): Financial assistance from the Social Security Administration for disabled people with income below a certain level (chapter 18).

Supplements: Nutritional drinks that are rich in calories, protein, and vitamins are called supplements. These drinks, such as Ensure, can help a person maintain weight or put on weight (chapter 4).

Sustiva (also called efavirenz): A non-nucleotide reverse transcriptase inhibitor HIV treatment (chapter 6).

T-20: See *Fuzeon.*

Tenofovir: See *Viread.*

Thalidomide: An oral medication used to treat sores thought to be caused by HIV. The sores may be on the genitals or in the mouth or esophagus. Thalidomide can cause severe birth defects, so at least two forms of birth control should be used by women with the ability to become pregnant who are taking thalidomide (chapter 8).

Therapeutic drug monitoring: Checking blood levels of specific HIV treatments to be sure they are adequate (chapter 6).

3TC: See *Epivir.*

Thrush (also called oral candidiasis): A yeast infection of the mouth that can extend down the esophagus (the tube connecting the mouth to the stomach). Usually thrush looks like cottage cheese in the mouth. Thrush can cause mouth pain and difficulty eating and swallowing (chapter 4).

Toxoplasmosis: Infection of the brains of people with HIV by a parasite. Symptoms include weakness in one or more limbs and seizures (convulsions). The diagnosis of toxoplasmosis requires either a CAT scan or MRI study of the head (chapter 4).

Tramadol: See *Ultram.*

Trichomoniasis: A vaginal infection that can cause a bothersome, heavy discharge that may be greenish or yellow and itching or soreness (chapter 8).

Triglycerides: A form of fat in the bloodstream. Their levels may increase with certain HIV treatments, increasing the risk for heart disease or pancreatitis. People with high triglyceride levels may require medical treatment (chapter 13).

Trimethoprim/sulfamethoxazole: See *Bactrim.*

Trizivir: A combination of Retrovir, Epivir, and Ziagen (chapter 6).

Tubal ligation: A minor surgical procedure often referred to as "tying the tubes." Tubal ligation effectively prevents pregnancy (chapter 10).

Tuberculosis (TB): A disease caused by *Mycobacterium tuberculosis*, which generally causes lung infections. People with TB lung infections who are not treated can transmit the infection to others by breathing or coughing the bacteria into the air that others inhale. Symptoms of active tuberculosis include high fever, weight loss, cough, and shortness of breath (chapter 10).

Ultram (also called tramadol): A weak, short-acting opioid medication prescribed to treat pain. It is a good choice for people who have kidney or liver problems and whose pain is not severe.

Uterine fibroids: Growths in the uterus that may also be called fibroid tumors. They are not cancerous.

Uterus (also called the womb): A muscular sac in the lower abdomen that protects and holds a growing baby during pregnancy. When a woman is not pregnant, her uterine lining is normally refreshed every month as part of the natural menstrual cycle.

Vasectomy: A minor surgical procedure performed on men as a method of permanent birth control. The vasectomy prevents the sperm from coming out with the semen (chapter 10).

Vaginal yeast infection (also called *Candida* vaginitis): A yeast infection can cause symptoms of vaginal itching, burning, and soreness and may be accompanied by a white vaginal discharge (chapter 8).

Valcyte (also called valganciclovir): A treatment for cytomegalovirus (CMV). Valcyte is a pill that is given initially twice daily and then only once daily after the first three weeks.

Valganciclovir: See *Valcyte.*

Valtrex (also called valcyclovir): A medication given by mouth to treat herpes infections, a cause of genital sores (chapter 8).

Vfend (also called voriconazole): A strong anti-fungal treatment that may be effective against infections such as *Candida* or cryptococcal meningitis, which are resistant to Diflucan (chapter 4).

Videx (also called didanosine or ddI): A nucleoside reverse transcriptase inhibitor HIV treatment (chapter 6).

Viracept (also called nelfinavir): A protease inhibitor HIV treatment (chapter 6).

Viral load tests: These tests measure how much HIV is in a person's blood. There are two types of viral load tests. One test looks for "branched chain DNA (bDNA)"; the other is a quantitative HIV RNA-PCR. Both measure genetic material of the virus and show the concentration of HIV present in the blood (chapter 3).

Virammune (also called nevirapine): A non-nucleotide reverse transcriptase inhibitor HIV treatment (chapter 6).

Viread (also called tenofovir): A nucleotide reverse transcriptase inhibitor HIV treatment (chapter 6).

Vistide (also called cidofovir): A medication given through the vein to treat cytomegalovirus infections (CMV).

Voriconazole: See *Vfend.*

Western blot test: Test used to confirm ELISA test results that indicate a person has been infected with HIV (chapter 1).

Zalcitibine: See *Hivid.*

Zerit (also called stavudine or d4T): A nucleoside reverse transcriptase inhibitor HIV treatment (chapter 6).

Ziagen (also called abacavir): A nucleoside reverse transcriptase inhibitor HIV treatment (chapter 6).

Zidovudine: See *Retrovir.*

Zithromax (also called azithromycin): An antibiotic medication prescribed for various bacterial infections. It is often used to protect people with low CD4 cell counts against *Mycobacterium avium-intracellulare* complex (MAC) or to treat MAC (chapter 4).

Zovirax (also called acyclovir): A treatment for a herpes infection, one cause of genital sores. The medication can be given by mouth, applied as a topical cream, or injected into the vein (chapter 8).

Key References

The following are scientific references that were the source for much of the information in the chapters. You may be able to access the medical journals only in a medical school library, but all Web site references should be readily available.

INTRODUCTION. WOMEN AND THE HIV/AIDS EPIDEMIC

Centers for Disease Control. *Morb Mort Wkly Rept* 50 (2001): 429–45.
Centers for Disease Control Summary of all the reports on HIV and AIDS at www.cdc.gov/mmwr/hiv_aids20.html.

CHAPTER 1. TESTING FOR HIV

Anderson, J., ed. "A Guide to the clinical care of women with HIV." U.S. Department of Health and Human Services, Health Resources Services Administration at www.hrsa.gov/hab.
Byland, D. J., U. H. Ziegner, and D. G. Hooper. "Review of testing for human immunodeficiency virus." *Clin Lab Med* 12 (1992): 305–33.
Celum, C., and S. Buchbinder. "Counseling and testing for HIV infection." In K. K. Holmes, P. F. Sparling, P. A. Mardh et al., eds. *Sexually Transmitted Diseases*. New York: McGraw-Hill, 1999.
Centers for Disease Control. "Interpretation and use of the Western blot assay for serodiagnosis of human immunodeficiency virus type 1 infections." *Morb Mort Wkly Rep* 38 (1989): (S-7): 1–7.

CHAPTER 3. HIV, THE IMMUNE SYSTEM, AND MONITORING TESTS

Cao, Y., I. L. Qin, J. Zhang, J. Safrit, and D. D. Ho. "Virologic and immunologic characterization of long-term survivors of human immunodeficiency virus type 1 infection." *N Engl J Med* 332 (1995): 201–8.

Fauci, A. S., G. Pantaleo, S. Stanley, and D. Weissman. "Immunopathogenic mechanisms of HIV infection." *Ann Intern Med* 124 (1996): 654–63.

Hessol, N. A., A. R. Lifson, and G. W. Rutherford. "Natural history of human immunodeficiency virus infection and key predictors of HIV disease progression." *AIDS Clin Rev* (1989): 69–93.

Kahn, J. O., and B. D. Walker. "Acute human immunodeficiency virus type 1 infection." *N Engl J Med* 339 (1998): 33–39.

Mellors, J. W., A. Munoz, J. V. Giogi et al. "Plasma viral load and CD4 + lymphocytes as prognostic markers of HIV-infection." *Ann Intern Med* 126 (1997): 946–54.

Moore, R. S., L. Cheever, J. C. Keruly, and R. D. Chaisson. "Lack of sex difference in CD4 to HIV-1 RNA viral load ratio." *Lancet* 353 (1999): 464.

CHAPTER 4. RECOGNIZING SYMPTOMS AND PREVENTING COMPLICATIONS

Carpenter, C. J. C., K. H. Mayer, M. D. Stein, B. D. Leibman, A. Fisher, and T. C. Fiore. "Human immunodeficiency virus infection in North American women: Experience with 200 cases and a review of the literature." *Medicine* 70 (1991): 307–25.

Centers for Disease Control. "Guidelines for preventing opportunistic infections among persons infected with human immunodeficiency virus—2002 recommendations of the US Public Health Service and the Infectious Diseases Society of America." MMWR No. RR-8 (2002): 51.

———. "Revision of the CDC surveillance case definition for acquired immunodeficiency syndrome." *Morb Mort Wkly Rep* 36 (1987): 3S–11S.

Clark, R. A., W. Brandon, J. Dumestre, and C. Pindaro. "Clinical manifestations of infection with the human immunodeficiency virus in women in Louisiana." *Clin Infect Dis* 17 (1993): 173–77.

Fleming, P. J., C. A. Ciesielski, R. H. Byers, K. G. Castro, and R. L. Berkelman. "Gender differences in reported AIDS-indicative diagnoses." *J Infect Dis* 168 (1993): 61–67.

CHAPTER 5. HEPATITIS AND THE LIVER

"NIH Consensus Development Conference Statement: Management of Hepatitis C." (June 10–12, 2002): 19(1) at http://consensus.nih.gov/cons/116/116cdc_statement.htm.

Centers for Disease Control. "Recommendations for prevention and control of HCV infection and HCV-related chronic disease." *Morb Mort Wkly Rep* 47 (1998): 1–39.

Heathcote, E. J., M. L. Shiffman, W. T. Cooksley et al. "Peginterferon alfa-2a in patients with chronic hepatitis C and cirrhosis. *N Engl J Med* 343 (2000): 1673–80.

Lok, A. S. "Chronic hepatitis B." *N Engl J Med* 346 (2002): 1682–83.

Soriano, V., M. Sulkowski, C. Bergin et al. "Care of patients with chronic hepatitis C and HIV co-infection: Recommendations from the HIV-HCV International Panel." *AIDS* 16 (2002): 813–28.

CHAPTER 6. TREATMENTS FOR HIV

Bersoff-Matcha, S. J., W. C. Miller, J. A. Aberg et al. "Sex difference in nevirapine rash." *Clin Infect Dis* 32 (2001): 124–29.

Carpenter, C., D. Cooper, M. Fischl et al. "Antiretroviral therapy in adults: Updated recommendations of the International AIDS Society—USA Panel." *JAMA* 283 (2000): 381–90.

Centers for Disease Control. "U.S. Public Health Service Task Force recommendations for use of antiretroviral drugs in pregnant HIV-infected women for maternal health and interventions to reduce perinatal HIV transmission in the United States." *Morb Mort Wkly Rep.*

Dong, K. L., L. L. Bausserman, M. M. Flynn et al. "Changes in body habitus and serum lipid abnormalities in HIV-positive women on highly active antiretroviral therapy." *J Acquir Immune Defic Synd* 21 (1999): 107–13.

Gazzard, B., and G. Moyle. "1998 Revision to the British HIV Association guidelines for antiretroviral treatment of HIV seropositive individuals." *Lancet* 352 (1998): 314–16.

Gervasoni, C., A. L. Ridolfo, G. Trifiro et al. "Redistribution of body fat in HIV-infected women undergoing combination antiretroviral therapy." *AIDS* 13 (1999): 465–71.

Hadigan, C., K. Miller, C. Corcoran, E. Anderson, N. Basgoz, and S. Grinspoon. "Fasting hyperinsulinemia and changes in regional body composition in human immunodeficiency virus-infected women." *J Clin Endocrinol Metab* 84 (1999): 1932–37.

National Guidelines available at http://aidsinfo.nih.gov/guidelines or www.cdcnpin.org.

Powderly, W. G. "Sorting through confusing messages: The art of HAART." *J Acquir Immune Defic Synd* 31 (2002): S3–9.

Schambelan, M., C. A. Benson, A. Carr, J. S. Currier et al. "Management of metabolic complications associated with antiretroviral therapy for HIV infection: Recommendations of an International AIDS Society—USA panel." *J Acquir Immune Def Synd* 31 (2002): 257–70.

Toumala, R. E., et al. "Antiretroviral therapy during pregnancy and the risk of an adverse outcome." *N Engl J Med* 346 (2002): 1863–70.

Watts, H. D. "Management of HIV in pregnancy." *N Engl J Med* 346 (2002): 1879–91.

Wit, F. W., G. J. Weverling, J. Weel, S. Jurriaans, and J. M. Lange. "Incidence of and risk factors for severe hepatotoxicity associated with antiretroviral combination therapy." *J Infect Dis* 186 (2002): 23–31.

CHAPTER 7. PROTECTING YOURSELF AND OTHERS

Centers for Disease Control. "Public Health Service guidelines for the management of health-care worker exposures to HIV and recommendations for post exposure prophylaxis." *Mort Morb Wkly Report* 47, RR-7 (1998): 1–34.

Glaser, A. "Emergency postcoital contraception." *N Engl J Med* 337 (1997): 1058–64.

Kahn, J. O., J. N. Martin, M. E. Roland et al. "Feasibility of post exposure prophylaxis (PEP) against human immunodeficiency virus infection after sexual or injection drug use exposure: The San Francisco PEP study." *J Infect Dis* 183 (2001): 707–14.

Uckin, F., and O. Druz. "Prophylactic contraceptives for HIV/AIDS." *Human Reproduction Update* 5 (1999): 506–14.

CHAPTER 8. GYNECOLOGIC INFECTIONS AND SEXUALLY TRANSMITTED DISEASES

Anderson, J., R. A. Clark, H. Watts et al. "Idiopathic genital ulcers in women infected with human immunodeficiency virus." *J Acquir Immune Def Synd* 13 (1996): 343–47.

Barbosa, C., M. Macasaet, S. Brockmann, M. F. Sierra, Z. Xia, and A. Duerr. "Pelvic inflammatory disease and human immunodeficiency virus disease." *Obstet Gynecol* 89 (1997): 65–70.

Bukesi, E. A., C. R. Cohen, C. E. Stevens et al. "Effects of human immunodeficiency virus infection on microbial origins of pelvic inflammatory disease and on efficacy of ambulatory oral therapy." *Am J Obstet Gynecol* 18 (1999): 1374–81.

Centers for Disease Control. "1998 Guidelines for Treatment of Sexually Transmitted Diseases." *Morb Mort Wkly Report* 47 (1997): 1–118.

———. "Sexually Transmitted Diseases Treatment Guidelines 2002." *Morb Mort Wkly Rep* 51 (2002): 1–80.

Cohen, C. R., S. Sinei, M. Reilly et al. "Effect of human immunodeficiency virus infection upon acute salpingitis in a laparoscopic study." *J Infect Dis* 178 (1998): 1352–58.

Greenblatt, R. M., P. Bacchetti, S. Barkan et al. "Lower genital tract infections among HIV-infected and high-risk uninfected women." *Sex Trans Dis* 26 (1999): 143–51.

Hoegsberg, B., O. Abulafia, A. Sedlis, J. Feldman, D. DesJalais, S. Landesman, and H. Minkoff. "Sexually transmitted diseases and human immunodeficiency virus infection among women with pelvic inflammatory disease." *Am J Obstet Gynecol* 163 (1990): 1135–39.

Imam, N., C. C. Carpenter, K. H. Mayer, A. Fisher, M. Stein, and S. B. Danforth. "Hierarchical pattern of mucosal candida infections in HIV-seropositive women." *Am J Med* 89 (1990): 142–46.

Irwin, K. L., A. C. Moorman, M. J. O'Sullivan et al. "Influence of human immunodeficiency virus infection." *Obstet Gynecol* 95 (2000): 525–34.

Jamieson, D. J., A. Duerr, R. S. Klein et al. "Longitudinal analysis of bacterial vaginosis: Findings from the HIV epidemiology research study." *Obstet Gynecol* 98 (2001): 656–63.

Kamenga, M., K. M. DeCock, M. E. St. Louis et al. "The impact of human immunodeficiency virus infection on pelvic inflammatory disease: A case-control study in Abidjan, Ivory Coast." *Am J Obstet Gynecol* 172 (1995): 919–25.

Schuman, P., L. Capps, G. Peng et al. "Weekly fluconazole for the prevention of mucosal candidiasis in women with HIV infection." *Ann Intern Med* 126 (1997): 689–96.

Sewell, C. A., and J. R. Anderson. "Cytomegalovirus disease in the lower genital tract." *AIDS Patient Care STDs* 15 (2001): 459–62.

Sobel, J. D. "Vaginitis." *N Engl J Med* 337 (1997): 1896–903.

Warren, D., R. S. Klein, J. Sobel et al. "A multicenter study of bacterial vaginosis in women with or at risk for human immunodeficiency virus infection." *Infect Dis Obstet Gynecol* 9 (2001): 133–41.

CHAPTER 9. HUMAN PAPILLOMAVIRUS INFECTIONS, GENITAL WARTS, AND ABNORMAL PAP SMEARS

Ahdieh, L., R. S. Klein, R. Burk et al. "Prevalence, incidence, and type-specific persistence of human papillomavirus in human immunodeficiency virus (HIV)-positive and HIV-negative women." *J Infect Dis* 184 (2001): 682–90.

Centers for Disease Control. "Risk for cervical disease in HIV infected women New York City." *Morb Mort Wkly Rep* 39 (1990): 846–49.

Ho, G. Y. F., R. Bierman, L. Beardsley, C. H. Chang, and R. D. Burk. "Natural history of cervicovaginal papillomavirus infection in young women." *N Engl J Med* 338 (1998): 423–28.

Koutsky, L. A., K. K. Holmes, C. W. Critchlow, C. E. Stevens, J. Paavonen, A. M.

Beckmann, T. A. DeRouen, D. A. Galloway, D. Bernon, and N. B. Kiviat. "A cohort study of the risk of cervical intraepithelial neoplasia grade 2 or 3 in relation to papillomavirus infection." *N Engl J Med* 327 (1992): 1272–78.

Kurman, R. J., D. E. Henson, A. Herbst, K. L. Nollar, and M. H. Schiffman. "Interim guidelines for management of abnormal cervical cytology." *JAMA* 271 (1994): 1866–69.

Maiman, M., D. H. Watts, J. Andersen, P. Clax, M. Merino, and M. A. Kendall. "Vaginal 5-fluorouracil for high-grade dysplasia in human immunodeficiency virus infection: A randomized trial." *Obstet Gynecol* 94 (1999): 954–61.

Massad, L. S., K. A. Reister, K. M. Anastos et al. "Prevalence and predictors of squamous cell abnormalities in Papanicolaou smears from women infected with HIV." *J Acquir Immune Defic Synd* 21 (1999): 33–41.

Robinson, W. R., J. Andersen, T. M. Darragh, M. A. Kendall, R. A. Clark, and M. Maiman. "Isotretinoin for low-grade cervical dysplasia in human immunodeficiency virus-infected women." *Obstet Gynecol* 99 (2002): 777–84.

Sun, W., L. Kuhn, T. V. Ellerbrock, M. A. Chiasson, T. J. Bush, and T. Wright. "Human papillomavirus infection in women infected with human immunodeficiency virus." *N Engl J Med* 337 (1997):1343–49.

CHAPTER 10. CONSIDERING PREGNANCY AND BIRTH CONTROL

"A Guide to the Clinical Care of Women with HIV" at www.hrsa.gov/hab

Al-Chan, A., J. Colon, and A. Bardeguez. "Assisted reproductive technology for men and women infected with HIV." *Clin Infect Dis* 36 (2003): 195–200.

Centers for Disease Control. "1998 guidelines for treatment of sexually transmitted diseases." *MMWR* 47, RR-1 (1998): 1–116.

———. "Sexually transmitted diseases treatment guidelines 2002." *Morbid Mortal Wkly Rep* 51 (2002): 1–80.

Lyerly, A. D., and J. Anderson. "HIV and assisted reproduction: Reconsidering evidence, reframing ethics." *Fert Steril* 75 (2001): 843–58.

CHAPTER 11. PREGNANCY

Centers for Disease Control. "2001 USPHS/IDSA guidelines for the prevention of opportunistic infections with persons infected with human immunodeficiency virus."

———. "Public Health Service Task Force Recommendations for Use of Antiretroviral Drugs in Pregnant HIV-1-Infected Women for Maternal Health and Interventions to Reduce Perinatal HIV-1-Transmission in the United States" at http://aidsinfo.nih.gov/guidelines

Connor, E. M., R. S. Sperling, R. Gelber et al. "Reduction of maternal-infant transmission of human immunodeficiency virus type 1 with zidovudine treatment." *N Engl J Med* 331 (1994): 1173–80.

Landesman, S. H., L. A. Kalish, D. N. Burns et al. "Obstetrical factors and the transmission of human immunodeficiency virus type 1 from mother to child: The Women and Infants Transmission Study." *N Engl J Med* 334 (1996): 1617–23.

Watts, D. H., J. S. Lambert, E. Stiehm. "Complications according to mode of delivery among HIV-infected women with CD4 cell counts of less than or equal to 500." *Am J Obstet Gynecol* 183 (2000): 100–107.

CHAPTER 12. MENSTRUAL PERIODS

Clark, R. A., and R. Bessinger. "Clinical manifestations and predictors of survival among older women infected with HIV." *J Acquir Immune Defic Synd* 15 (1997): 341–45.

Clark, R. A., S. Cohn, C. Jarek, K. S. Craven, C. Lyons, M. Jacobson, and L. Kamemoto. "Perimenopausal symptomatology among HIV-infected women at least 40 years of age." *J Acquir Immune Defic Synd* 22 (1999): 408–9.

Glazier, M. G., and M. A. Bowman. "A review of the evidence for the use of phytoestrogens as replacement for traditional estrogen replacement therapy." *Arch Intern Med* 161 (2001): 1161–72.

Manson, J. E., and K. A. Martin. "Postmenopausal hormone-replacement therapy." *N Engl J Med* 345 (2001): 34–-40.

Nelson, H. D. "Assessing benefits and harms of hormone replacement therapy." *JAMA* 288 (2002): 882–84.

Nelson, H. D., L. L. Humphrey, P. Nygren, S. M. Teutsch, and J. D. Allan. "Postmenopausal hormone replacement therapy." *JAMA* 288 (2002): 872–81.

Olive, D. L., and L. B. Schwarz. "Endometriosis." *N Engl J Med* 328 (1993): 1759–69.

CHAPTER 13. BREAST HEALTH, BONE HEALTH, AND HEART HEALTH

Cadarette, S. M., S. B. Jaglal, T. M. Murray et al. "Evaluation of decision rules for referring women for bone densitormetry by DEXA." *JAMA* 286 (2001): 57–63.

Guth, A. A. "Breast cancer and HIV: What do we know?" *Am Surg* 65 (1999): 209–11.

McDermott, A. Y., A. Shevitz, T. Knox et al. "Effect of highly active antiretroviral therapy on fat, lean, and bone mass in HIV-seropositive men and women." *Am J Clin Nutr* 74 (2001): 679–86.

National Cholesterol Education Program. "Second report of the expert panel on detection, evaluation, and treatment of high blood cholesterol in adults (Adult Treatment Panel II)." *Circulation* 89 (1994): 1329–445.

———. "Third report of the expert panel on detection, evaluation, and treatment of high blood cholesterol in adults (Adult Treatment Panel III)." *JAMA* 285 (2001): 2486–97.

Pernerstorfer-Schoen, H., B. Jilma, A. Perschler et al. "Sex differences in HAART-associated dyslipidaemia." *AIDS* 15 (2001): 725–34.

Schambelan, M., C. A. Benson, A. Carr et al. "Management of metabolic complications associated with antiretroviral therapy for HIV infection: Recommendations of an International AIDS Society—USA panel." *J Acquir Immune Defic Synd* 31 (2002): 257–67.

Tebas, P., W. G. Powderly, S. Claxton et al. "Accelerated bone mineral loss in HIV-infected patients receiving potent antiretroviral therapy." *AIDS* 14 (2000): F63–7.

CHAPTER 14. ALCOHOL DEPENDENCE, DRUG ADDICTION, AND TREATMENT

Anderson, J., ed. "A guide to the clinical care of women with HIV" at www .hrsa.gov/hab.

Mathias, R. "Blood pressure medication may improve cocaine treatment results in patients with severe withdrawal symptoms" at www.drugabuse.gov/ NIDANotes/NNVo116N6/Blood.html.

CHAPTER 15. INTIMATE PARTNER VIOLENCE AND ABUSE

Cohen, M., C. Deamant, S. Barkan et al. "Domestic violence and childhood sexual abuse in HIV-infected and women at risk for HIV." *Am J Public Health* 90 (2000): 560–65.

Edelson, J. L. "The overlap between child maltreatment and woman battering." *Violence Against Women* 5, no. 2 (February 1999): 134–54.

Evans, P. *The verbally abusive relationship: How to recognize it and how to respond.* Holbrook, MA: Adams Media Corporation, 1999.

McCauley, J., D. E. Kern, K. Kolodner et al. "The 'Battering Syndrome': Prevalence and clinical characteristics of domestic violence in primary care internal medicine practices." *Ann Intern Med* 123 (1995): 737–46.

Miller, M. S. *No visible wounds.* New York: Ballantine Books, 1996.

Rennison, C. M., and S. Welchans. *Intimate Partner Violence, Bureau of Justice Statistics Special Report.* Washington, D.C.: U.S. Department of Justice, 2000.

CHAPTER 16. MANAGING YOUR FEELINGS

Ferrando, S. J., J. G. Rabkin, G. M. de Moore, and R. Rabkin. "Antidepressant treatment of depression in HIV-seropositive women." *J Clin Psychiatry* 60 (1999): 741–46.

"Psychiatric aspects of HIV care." *AIDS Clinical Care* (2001): 101–8.

Whooley, M. A., and G. E. Simon. "Managing depression in medical outpatients." *N Engl J Med* 343 (2000): 1942–49.

CHAPTER 17. CHRONIC PAIN, PALLIATIVE CARE, AND HOSPICE

Hoffmann, D. E., and A. J. Tarzian. "The girl who cried pain: A bias against women in the treatment of pain." *J of Law, Medicine and Ethics* 29 (2001): 13–27.

CHAPTER 18. PLANNING FOR THE FUTURE

McGovern, T. "Legal issues affecting women with HIV." In *The Medical Management of AIDS in Women*. New York: Wiley-Liss, 1997.

Index

abacavir. *See* Ziagen
abuse of women, 16, 265; effect on
 children, 202–4; by intimate partner, 199–202; making a safety
 plan, 206–7; people who are
 abusers, 202; planning escape,
 207–8; post-traumatic stress disorder and, 222; reasons women feel
 they cannot leave, 205–6; recognition of, 200–201; resources for
 help and shelter, 210–15; risks of
 escape, 108–9; staying with
 abusers, 202–4
acyclovir (Zovirax), 120, 291
addiction, 187–91, 265; to analgesics,
 227, 228; vs. drug dependence,
 228; of newborn, 135; pain control
 in people with, 236–37; treatment
 of, 192–98
adefovir (Hepsera), 275; for hepatitis B,
 66–67
adjusting to life with HIV, 7, 56
adolescents: research with, 253; understanding of illness by, 18–19
advance directives, 244–45
Advil, 45, 61, 230
African-American women, 3
Agenerase (amprenavir), 80, 82–84,
 149, 265; food requirements and
 dosing of, 85; interaction with
 birth control pills, 95–96; in pregnancy, 135; side effects of, 91, 92

AIDS, 2, 265; difference from HIV
 infection, 48; progression from
 HIV infection to, 33–36
AIDS Clinical Trials Group, 265–6
Aid to Families with Dependent
 Children, 243
alcoholism, 187, 191–92, 266; treatment of, 197
Aldara cream, 125, 266
alendronate (Fosamax), 182, 274
Aleve, 45, 46, 61, 230
l-alpha-acetylmethadol (LAAM),
 195
alprazolam (Xanax), 223, 225
Alzheimer's disease, 172, 266
Ambien (zolpidem), 223–25
amenorrhea, 165, 167, 266
amitriptyline. *See* Elavil
amphotericin, 46, 266
amprenavir. *See* Agenerase
anabolic treatments, 47, 164, 266
Anadrol (oxymetholone), 47
Anafranil (clomipramine), 218–19
analgesics, 229–37; addiction to, 227,
 228; for headache, 234–35; for
 people addicted to drugs, 236–37.
 See also pain
anemia, 42–43, 90, 266
anergy, 55, 266
anger, 14
anovulation, 164, 166
Antabuse (disulfiram), 197

antibiotics, 43, 266; prophylactic, 56–57

antibodies, 9–10, 31–32, 267; against hepatitis B, 64; in infants, 12

antidepressants, 217–21

antigen, 267; hepatitis B, 64

Antiretroviral Pregnancy Registry, 97, 136

antiretrovirals, 29–30, 72–99, 267; after unprotected sex, 108; for antiretroviral-experienced patients, 87–89, 267; for antiretroviral-naive patients, 79–87, 267; classes of, 73; cocktail of, 78, 270; drug interactions with, 69, 94–96, 196, 219–20, 222; food requirements and dosing of, 84–86; in future, 98; intensification of, 88, 277; keeping track of, 79–81, 261; once-daily therapy with, 84; in pregnancy, 78, 83, 96–97, 135–36, 155–60; recommended regimens of, 81–83; side effects of, 89–94; starting, 74–78; stopping, 98; therapeutic drug monitoring of, 89, 288; viral resistance to, 74–75, 88–89, 158. *See also* medications

anxiety disorders, 221–23

anxiolytics, 222–23, 267; interaction with Norvir, 222, 225

ASCUS (atypical squamous cells of undetermined significance), 126, 267

aspirin, 231–32

astemizole, 96

asymptomatic period, 32–33, 35

atazanavir. *See* Reyataz

Ativan (lorazepam), 223, 225

atorvastatin (Lipitor), 185, 278

atovaquone (Mepron), 53, 56, 57, 279

atypical squamous cells of undetermined significance (ASCUS) on Pap smear, 126, 267

azithromycin (Zithromax), 52, 57, 117, 290–91

AZT. *See* Retrovir

bacterial vaginosis, 113–14, 267

Bactrim (trimethoprim/sulfamethoxazole), 53, 57, 267

basal temperature monitoring, 140–42

benzodiazepines, 197, 223, 224, 267

Biaxin (clarithromycin), 52, 56, 57, 267–68

biopsy, 268; breast, 179; cervical, 127; uterine, 166

birth control methods, 142–49; choosing among, 142–43; comparison of, 146–48; effectiveness for pregnancy prevention, 143–44; HIV infection and, 145–49; for prevention of sexually transmitted disease, 144; reversible, 145

birth control pills, 36, 143, 145–47, 166, 282; drug interactions with, 95–96

birth to HIV-positive mother, 154–55

bisphosphonates, 182, 268

black cohosh, 173

bleach for disinfection, 110–11

blinding in clinical trials, 258, 268

blood cell count, 26, 268

blood tests, 26, 268; for hepatitis B, 24, 63–65; for HIV, 9–15; for syphilis, 24, 121; for toxoplasmosis, 24

blue cohosh, 173

bone health, 180–82

bone pain, 229; control of, 230–31

boosted protease inhibitors, 84, 88, 95, 268

breast: fibroadenoma of, 180; fibrocystic disease of, 179, 274; lumps in, 179–80

breast biopsy, 179

breast cancer, 177–80

Emtriva (emtricitabine), 80, 82, 84; food requirements and dosing of, 85; for hepatitis B, 66; side effects of, 90

encephalitis, 51–52; *Toxoplasma*, 53–54, 288

endocrinology, 22

endometriosis, 168, 272

endometrium, 168, 272

endoscopy, 49, 273

enfuvirtide. *See* Fuzeon

entry inhibitors, 30, 273

eosinophilic folliculitis, 46, 273

epidemic of HIV/AIDS, 1–2

Epivir (lamivudine), 80–81, 84, 273; food requirements and dosing of, 85; for hepatitis B, 66; during labor, 158; for newborn, 158; side effects of, 90, 92; viral resistance to, 158

Epogen (erythromycin), 117

Ergotamine, 235

erythromycin (Epogen), 117

erythropoietin (Procrit), 43, 273

esophagitis, *Candida*, 48, 49, 268

esophagus, 49, 273

evening primrose oil, 168, 173

Evista (raloxifene), 182, 273

exercise, 181, 184

famciclovir (Famvir), 120, 273

family: informing of HIV diagnosis, 15–19

Famvir (famciclovir), 120, 273

fatigue, 44, 273

fat maldistribution, 92–93

Femring, 173, 273

fetal alcohol syndrome, 193, 273

fibroadenoma of breast, 180

fibrocystic breast disease, 179, 274

Flagyl (metronidazole), 114, 115, 274

Floxin (ofloxacin), 117–18

fluconazole. *See* Diflucan

fluoxetine (Prozac), 167, 218–19, 223

flurazepam (Dalmane), 224, 225

fluvoxamine (Luvox), 218–19

follicle stimulating hormone, 141, 165, 170, 274

folliculitis, eosinophilic, 46, 273

Food and Drug Administration (FDA), 97, 249, 251, 274

Fortivase (saquinavir), 80, 82–83, 274; food requirements and dosing of, 85; side effects of, 91, 92

Fosamax (alendronate), 182, 274

foscarnet (Foscavir), 51, 122

Foscavir (foscarnet), 51, 122

fractures, 180, 182

FTC. *See* Emtriva

5–FU (5–fluorouracil), 128

fusion inhibitors, 73, 80, 98, 274

Fuzeon (enfuvirtide), 80, 89, 98, 274; food requirements and dosing of, 85; side effects of, 91

gabapentin (Neurontin), 45, 229–30, 280

ganciclovir (Cytovene), 51, 122, 271

gemfibrozil (Lopid), 185, 278

General Public Assistance, 243

generic drug names, 5, 274

genital ulcers, 42, 48, 104, 105, 118, 275; in pregnancy, 152

genital warts, 123–25; in pregnancy, 152

genotype test, 86, 87, 275

glucose tolerance test, 161, 282

gonorrhea, 105, 116–18, 141, 275

Halcion, 96

headaches, 90–92, 229, 233–35

Health Insurance Portability and Accountability Act, 251

heart health, 182–85

hematology/oncology, 275

hepatitis, 60–71, 90, 92, 275; protecting liver in, 61–63; transmission of, 63; vaccines against, 61–62

hepatitis A, 60–62

starting HIV treatment, 86–87; for blood fat levels, 183–84; for hepatitis B, 63–65; for HIV, 9–15; for pregnancy, 150; in pregnancy, 160, 161; for syphilis, 121; tracking sheet for, 261

lactic acidosis, 69, 94, 278

lamivudine. *See* Epivir

laparoscopy, 168, 278

latex allergy, 106

legal preparations, 244–46

Lexiva (phosamprenavir), 80, 82, 84, 278; food requirements and dosing of, 85; side effects of, 91, 92

licorice, 173

life span, 241–42

Lipitor (atorvastatin), 185, 278

lipodystrophy, 92–93, 278–79

lipoprotein: high-density, 183, 275; low-density, 183–85, 278

liver protection, 61–63

liver transplantation, 70

living will, 244–45

Lomotil, 44

loop electrosurgical excision procedure, 127–28, 278

Lopid (gemfibrozil), 185, 278

lorazepam (Ativan), 223, 225

Lorcet, 231

Lortab, 189, 231

low-density lipoprotein cholesterol, 183–85, 278

Lunelle, 96, 143, 146, 147, 278

Luvox (fluvoxamine), 218–19

lymphadenopathy, 31, 44–45, 278

magnetic resonance imaging, 51–52, 54, 279

mammogram, 178

marijuana, 191

Marinol (dronabinol), 47–48, 279

medications: bringing to clinic visits, 25; clinical trials of, 248–59, 270;

liver damage from, 61; in pregnancy, 56, 78, 83, 96–97, 135; prophylactic, 56–57; refills of, 26. *See also* antiretrovirals

Megace, 47–48, 164, 167, 279

megestrol acetate. *See* Megace

meningitis, 279; cryptococcal, 49–50, 270–71

menopause, 164, 165, 169–71; hormone replacement therapy after, 171–73

menstrual periods, 163–74; cramps from, 168; HIV effects on, 168–69; premenstrual syndrome and, 167–68

Mepron (atovaquone), 53, 56, 57, 279

methadone: drug interactions with, 95, 196; for opioid addiction, 194–95

metronidazole (Flagyl), 114, 115, 274

Mevacor, 96

miconazole (Monistat), 115

Microsporidium, 44, 279

midazolam, 96

Midrin, 235

migraine, 233–35

milk thistle, 69–70

Mirena intrauterine device, 143, 145, 279

mirtazapine (Remeron), 218–19

Monistat (miconazole), 115

morphine, 228, 231, 233

Motrin, 61, 135, 166, 168, 230

mouth ulcers, 227

MS Contin, 189

mutations, 74–75, 86, 279–80

myalgia, 45, 90, 229, 280; medications for, 230–31

Mycelex, 46, 280

Mycobacterium avium-intracellulare complex (MAC), 44, 52–53, 57, 280

Mycobutin (rifabutin), 52–53, 57, 196, 280

myomectomy, 166

naloxone (Narcan), 195
Naprosyn, 135, 166, 168
Narcan (naloxone), 195
narcotics, 228. *See also* opioids
National Institutes of Health, 280
nausea, 90–92, 236
nefazodone (Serzone), 218–19, 223
nelfinavir. *See* Viracept
Neurontin (gabapentir), 45, 229–30, 280
neuropathy, 45, 90, 92, 229, 280; medications for, 229–30
nevirapine. *See* Virammune
New Drug Application, 257
nipple discharge, 178
non-nucleoside reverse transcriptase inhibitors (NNRTIs), 45, 73, 80–83, 280; side effects of, 90–92
nonoxynol-9, 105, 144, 280
non-progressors, 32–34, 280–81
non-steroidal anti-inflammatory drugs (NSAIDs), 45, 46, 281; liver damage from, 61, 62, 232; for menstrual problems, 166, 168; for pain, 230–33; in pregnancy, 135; side effects of, 234–35
Norplant, 143, 147, 164, 167, 281
Norpramin (desipramine), 218–19
nortriptyline (Pamelor), 218–19
Norvir (ritonavir), 80, 82–84, 281; drug interactions with, 196, 220, 222, 225; food requirements and dosing of, 85; protease inhibitors with, 89, 95; side effects of, 91, 92
nucleoside reverse transcriptase inhibitors, 73, 80–83, 281; side effects of, 90–92
nucleotide reverse transcriptase inhibitors, 73, 80, 281
numbness, 229–30
NuvaRING, 96, 143, 146, 147, 281
Nystatin, 46, 281

ofloxacin (Floxin), 117–18
opioids, 281; abuse of, 189–90; addiction to analgesics, 228; for pain, 45, 231–32; in pregnancy, 135; side effects of, 234–35; treatment of addiction to, 194–95
opportunistic processes, 48, 281–82
oral candidiasis, 42, 45–46, 49, 288
oral contraceptives, 36, 143, 145–47, 166, 282; drug interactions with, 95–96
oral sex, 105
Orasure test, 11
Ortho-evra, 96, 143, 146, 147, 282
osteonecrosis, 182, 282
osteoporosis, 173, 180–82, 282
ovulation, 137, 163–64, 282; HIV effects on, 168–69; timing of, 140–41
Oxandrin (oxandrolone), 47
oxandrolone (Oxandrin), 47
oxazepam (Serax), 223, 225
Oxycontin, 189
Oxyfast, 233
Oxyir, 233
oxymetholone (Anadrol), 47

pain, 226–39; barriers to control of, 228–29; bone or muscle, 229–31; control in people addicted to drugs, 236–37; diary of, 227–28; headaches, 90–92, 229, 233–35; medications for, 229–37; nerve, 229–30; nondrug therapies for, 237–38; pelvic, 168; visceral, 229, 231
palliative care, 238–39, 282
Pamelor (nortriptyline), 218–19
pancreatitis, 90, 92, 282
panic attacks, 221
Papanicolaou (Pap) smear, 25, 42, 116, 123–25, 282; atypical squamous cells of undetermined significance (ASCUS) on, 126, 267; cer-